DETERMINATION

DETERMINATION

RECAPTURING MY LIFE FROM LEUKEMIA

Deagara Robinson

Tate Publishing & *Enterprises*

Determination
Copyright © 2008 by Deagara Robinson. All rights reserved.

This title is also available as a Tate Out Loud product. Visit www.tatepublishing.com for more information.

No part of this publication may be reproduced, stored in a retrieval system or transmitted in any way by any means, electronic, mechanical, photocopy, recording or otherwise without the prior permission of the author except as provided by USA copyright law.

All Scripture quotations are taken from the *Holy Bible, New International Version* ®, Copyright © 1973, 1978, 1984 by International Bible Society. Used by permission of Zondervan Publishing House. All rights reserved.

This book is a true story. However, several names have been changed to protect the privacy of those involved.

Published by Tate Publishing & Enterprises, LLC
127 E. Trade Center Terrace | Mustang, Oklahoma 73064 USA
1.888.361.9473 | www.tatepublishing.com

Tate Publishing is committed to excellence in the publishing industry. The company reflects the philosophy established by the founders, based on Psalm 68:11,
"The Lord gave the word and great was the company of those who published it."

Book design copyright © 2008 by Tate Publishing, LLC. All rights reserved.
Cover design by Kellie Southerland
Interior design by Lance Waldrop

Published in the United States of America

ISBN: 978-1-60696-877-2
1. Biography & Autobiography / Medical
2. Biography & Autobiography / Religious
08.12.01

DEDICATION

I dedicate this book to my daughter and a new member to my family, Jayla Angelina Robinson, and every member of my family: Robinson, Roberson, Bennett, Edwards, Boswell, and Kivett, including my little sister, Stefanie K. Majors, who believes in my dreams and ideas and Callie M. Robinson, Lorenzo H. Robinson, Donny Roberson, Brett Barrett Hogan, and my great and grandparents—I'll always love and think of you.

ACKNOWLEDGMENTS

I would like to acknowledge the following people who have played a major role in my life. To my unrelated donor, thank you so much for being my best friend and having the courage to save my life. To my doctors, Dr. Monte Jones at Medical Center of Plano, Dr. Joseph W. Faye and Dr. Luis Pinero at Baylor University Medical Center, thank you so much for being so patient with me. To the brightest and smartest people that I have upmost respect for: Kay Reeves, Christina Mancuso, Mary Skelnik, Judy Bruton, Tyrone Bufford, Toni Keller, Amy Watts, Laura Brown, Russell Budd, and Fred Baron, thank you for being there during some the most difficult times of my life. To photo therapist, Christina Martinez and Christine Mullin at Texas Dermatology Associates at Baylor Medical Pavilion, thank you for being so sweet. Lorenzo Ferro Robinson, you are our father and mother's youngest child. You have kept us together as a family, and I'm so proud to call you're my little brother. You an example of the moral values our parents tried to install in us.

CHAPTERS

11	Introduction
15	Struggle
29	In Denial
51	My Battle to Live
69	Recapturing the Past
95	Putting My Life in Perspective
117	The Frustration of Understanding
135	My Own Fears and Trust Issues
147	It Was Time for Change
175	Facing My Fears
199	My Journal I
221	My Journal II
253	Conclusion

INTRODUCTION

I was very ignorant when it came to Leukemia, but once it affected my life, the reality came quickly that I had a fight on my hands. I never thought that something like this could've happen to me, but it did. Everything around me came to a complete stop because my life was on the line, but I also knew that it was really up to me to look at this situation in a positive way.

At first, I was too emotional to even talk to anyone about my prognoses because I was unwilling to accept that I was ever sick. But during that difficult time, it brought me closer to my spiritual beliefs. I realized now that there will always be trials and tribulations in my life and it was there to make me stronger and to teach me how to have more faith in God.

Yes, in the past, I had my own spiritual doubts, but not anymore, because I had to go through Leukemia for me to realize that I needed to put him first in my life. I was taught at a young age to respect my faith and that God does not give you something that you couldn't handle, but I knew I needed to learn how to let him fight my battles because I begin to realize that I actually don't have any control over certain things that goes on in my daily life.

Please understand that I don't wear my faith on my sleeves because I believe we have a right to choose what we want to believe in. It's not for me to judge others for their own personal beliefs. Some people are not going to see what you see or believe in what you believe in. I've learned to have an open mind so that I'm able to learn from anyone. I had to learn to take a good look at myself so that I could really find out what was best for me and be able to stand alone in what I believe in.

I always felt that God was with me during that difficult time of my life and he's still with me now. I don't worry as much as I did in the past because I know that God will work things out for me at the right time. I just needed to learn how to be patient. I realized that I have my own personal relationship with him and only he knows my heart and thoughts. Therefore, only he can judge me, and it's not my place to judge others or their own beliefs either.

During my hold turmoil, I learned how to be patient, which was one of my weaknesses. I didn't know *how* because, at the time, I was all over the place trying to resolve my problems and everyone else that has surrounded me too. It became to be so much for me that I didn't know how to relax or to focus on one thing at a time. I use to stress out on little things that weren't that important, but that changed quickly once my life was on the line. I begin to appreciate life more. Now I'm able to put things in a better perspective.

Most of my life, I always felt that I had to prove myself to others for acceptance rather than loving and accepting the person that I am. I had to learn what was going to make me happy because I never put myself first, and I had to find out the hard way. Once I was given a second chance in life, I learned how to put God first in my life and then me. But at the same time, I have a good heart. I care about people in general, and I felt that if I could share my story with others, maybe, it could help bring more knowledge and hope for someone else.

I hope by me writing this book I can bring a better understanding from my own experiences about this deadly disease and how it affects so many lives. There's still so much to be learn about Leukemia. I definitely don't have all the answers, but I do know how it is to have Leukemia. I know how it feels when you don't know if you're going to live or die and the frustration of sitting, waiting, wondering, and even hoping if they are able to locate a donor who was a match for my bone marrow.

I thought about others who are probably going through what I went through, who want to live but the only way to prolong their lives is a bone marrow transplant. I've learned that most minorities chances in finding a donor is very slim to none because the percentage are so low on the national registry. Believe me, I know because I was one of those minorities, but I was one of the lucky ones. I thank God for that.

If I can open at least one person's eyes to Leukemia, if he/she is able to relate to what I felt during that difficult time in my life, that would make me so happy. If by reading my story even one person is willing to join the registry to try to save another person's life, it would make this book worth writing. I've never met the person who saved my life, but she was willing to share a part of herself to save mine. I had some wonderful friends and doctors who were very supportive and played a major role in saving my life, and I'll never forget them. But there was one particular doctor who I thought at first didn't have good bedside manners because he didn't tell me what I wanted to hear. He knew that he couldn't promise me life, only hope. The last time I saw him, I made a promise that I would speak out about Leukemia but I knew that before I could do that I first had to learn how to love myself again.

There were many days I sat and thought about the journey it took me to get where I am today. It was the simple things in my life that I didn't appreciate before my illness. There were also memories in my past that I'd ran from but was able to put them in perspective. No matter what the consequences were, it happens and it was part of my life. How I dealt with it was the question.

I had a troubled life that I carried a lot of my pain within by distancing myself from others, but by writing this book, I'm now able to put closure to all the anger and fear I kept inside. I'm able to forgive others, including myself, because I realized my own faults throughout my journey. I've learned that with determination in any person can make a difference in their lives and in others too. I have accomplished so much in my life, and I will make mistakes. That's part of life, but I thank God, my friends, and family because without them I wouldn't be the person that I am now.

I can honestly say that by this process I've grown up a lot. I'm able to recognize my own mistakes and be responsible for them. I'm able to see things differently than before. I now realized that I will still have problems, but with determination, I know how to change various things into a positive like—things I really don't have control over—because I have enough faith to put my problems in God's hand.

STRUGGLE

I slowly stepped out the bathtub, as I grabbed a towel off the bar to dry off. I kneeled down to dry my legs when I noticed little flakes of my skin on the towel. At first, I thought it was a bad rash, but it was actually my *skin* pealing. I noticed a lot of discoloration all over my body especially on my legs. My doctor told me it would be months before I would see a difference in my skin after having a bone marrow transplant three months earlier.

I grabbed my bathrobe from behind the door as I walked into the dressing area. Before I wrapped my robe around me, I walked toward the mirror to get a better look at myself, which was something that I'd avoided for a very long time. However, I knew it was time for me to be honest and realistic about the hand that was dealt to me.

I didn't recognize myself anymore. I weighed 180 pounds. My face was dark, round, and very large from taking Prednisone for almost a year. As I stood there rubbing my head, I tried to feel if there was any hair growth. There was none. I touched my breast and stomach with the tips of my fingers where I noticed there were scabs of skin.

There was a Hickman implanted in the middle of my chest with three long white tubes folded together and taped with clear adhesive tape. The far right side of my chest had a lot of discoloration where the surgeon had surgically implanted a port inside of my chest. However, the catheter leaked during my chemotherapy, which was removed and replaced with the Hickman.

As I stood there looking at myself in the mirror, I begin to cry in the aftermath, side effects of chemotherapy and a bone marrow transplant. I stood there with tears pouring from my eyes as I tried to convince myself that there would be better days down the road for me. I just needed to learn to be patient. This was going to take time.

I put my robe on as I walked into the living room. I sat on the sofa as I went through my mail. As I fondle through my mail, I noticed a letter from my mother. I was hesitated to open it at first because we left our relationship on bad terms a month prior, but I went ahead and read it:

To my baby,
   I miss you very much. I don't care what you have said or done, I still love you because you're still my baby. I worry about you all the time. I forget where I'm going, or I forget where I live because my mind is on Dee all the time. God forgives us all for our sins. He's God and we are nothing but filthy rags, but he still loves us and I love you.
   Sign, Your Momma

I began crying again as I read her letter because I realized how much she really loved me. We had gotten into so many arguments when she was staying with me, which wasn't good for either of us. I knew within myself that I had to go through this difficult time alone. It was there to make me even stronger, but it was up to me to change my situation into something positive.

Nine months ago, I sent my daughter to Florida to live with her parental grandparents until I got better. I didn't want my child to see what I was about to go through because I felt that she wouldn't understand what was really happening to her mother. Even though she wasn't with me, she was my motivation to get better because I wanted my baby back with me.

I decided to move into a smaller and economize apartment, due to the fact that I was on disability and getting seventy percent of my income at the time. At first, I shared an apartment with my ex-boyfriend, but once I was diagnosed with Leukemia, everything between us changed quickly, and we decided to go our separate ways. It was for the best because God had opened my eyes to the true person he really was. It got to the point that I made him my focus when I should've been doing right in God's eyes first and then myself.

Every other day, I had to drive myself twenty miles back and forth from Plano to Dallas to see my oncologist at the Blood and Marrow Transplant Center at Baylor University Medical Center. I was still weak and under doctors' care after my bone marrow procedure, but I knew if I wanted to get better, I had to go in to see my doctor.

Whenever I arrived at the center, I would signed in up front before I sat and waited with the other patients in the waiting area before my name was called back to the lab to get my blood drawn for testing before I could see my doctor.

Once the lab technician called me into the lab, I would sit at this desk and watch as the technician drew my blood from one of my arms to test to see if my white blood count was still normal.

Afterward, I went back out front where I sat and waited until one of the nurses called my name so that I could visit with my doctor. The nurse always took my weight before assigning a patient's room. I would sit nervously as I waited for my doctor to walk through the door to discuss the lab results.

After meeting with my doctor and the results looked fine, I would normally go home, but if the result showed low in my red blood counts or my platelets were low, I had to stay for blood or platelet transfusion. They would set me up in one of there small cubical that was section off with a recliner and television attached to the arm of the chair and very long curtains to divide each section for little privacy. Before the transfusion took place, the nurse always provided me two Benadryl capsules to relax me before the transfusion. I watched as the nurse hooked my IV onto my Hickman line.

On one particular day, after visiting my doctor, I had to stay for a platelet transfusion. I sat in one of the cubical at the far end of the room as I glanced at the walls thinking about my life in general. As I looked up, I glanced across the room where I notice a man sitting across the room in one of the cubical facing me as the nurse was setting him up for a transfusion too. We made eye contact and smiled at one another, but soon, I went back looking at the wall, thinking how alone I was after my mother left.

The nurse came back over where I was sitting to check to see if I was okay and if I needed anything. "How are we doing?" the nurse asked. Is everything okay?"

"Yes," I said.

"How you're feeling?"

"I'm feeling fine, thanks for asking."

"You see the gentlemen sitting across the room from you?" she asked. I looked over where she was pointing.

"Yea," I said.

"Well, he wanted me to tell you that the two of you were going to beat this."

"Oh…really. That was nice." I looked over at him. As we made eye contact again, I smiled at him as he smiled back at me.

After the bone marrow procedure, I was prescribed many medications, which had various side effects. My hands shook like crazy to the point that I scribbled whenever I had to write or drive myself to the hospital. Sometimes, I actually had to hold onto the steering wheel really tight because my hands shocked so badly.

Whenever I had to pick up my medication, one pharmacist asked me how I was getting to the Bone Marrow Center. I told her that I drove myself to the hospital. She was amazed due to all the medication they prescribed me. She said she couldn't have done it, but I knew where my strength was coming from.

Once I provided the pharmacist my prescriptions, I sat and waited even though there were others ahead of me. I had time on my hands, plus I didn't have anywhere to rush off to. While I waited, I thought about the day that changed my life forever. I was so grateful that I was given a second chance in life, but I also realized that I had changed for the best.

August 17, 1997, is a date that I'll never forget! I was at work as I rushed into the firm's kitchen to fix myself a quick lunch before I went to my doctor's appointment for the second time. The kitchen was lined with people who were also waiting to put their food in the microwave. As I stood there in a deep thought, I was trying to figure out the reason I was so tired all the time and why I was running a high fever.

Earlier that week, my doctor prescribed me antibiotics, but it had no effect on my symptoms. I had to set up another doctor's appointment because this time my fever was up to 102 degrees and my ears were aching a lot, which I thought was very strange because I never had problems with my ears before. I was also so tired that I had no energy to even get dressed for work in the morning. I had to lie across the bed for ten minutes just so that I could build enough strength to get ready for work that day.

When I went in this time to see my doctor, who suggested they do blood work to check to see if something serious was going on. She too was puzzled as to why the antibiotic she had prescribed me wasn't relieving my symptoms. She thought that there was a chance I might be an anemic, but she wanted to first wait until the results came back from the lab to get an accurate diagnosis.

I had to reschedule to come back in to see her within a couple of days once the results came back from the lab. She also suggested that I needed to stay at home until my result was back in due to the fact that my fever was very high and it could also be contagious. I called my job and explained the situation to my manager.

A couple of days later, as I walked into the doctor's office, I noticed that there were a lot of people in the waiting room. I went up to the glass window where the receptionist was sitting to let her know that I was here to see Dr. Thompson. She asked me to sign in and to have a seat out in the waiting area and they should be calling me to the back soon.

As I looked out into the waiting room, I didn't know where to sit because the room was packed with people waiting to see their doctors. I noticed there was a seat in the corner by the front door. I sat down as I placed my purse on the floor next to my chair. I walked over to the table to select a magazine to read as I waited.

I begin to thumb through the magazine as I tried to find an interesting article to read while I waited. I felt that I would probably be sitting there for a while. As I began to read, the door slightly open as a nurse stood with a file in her hand. It seems like everyone who was waiting to see their doctors sat up in their seats once they saw her.

"Is there a De—agara?" I looked up because I knew she was trying to pronounce my name. A lot of people had a very difficult time pronouncing my name at first so I knew right off that she was looking for me.

"Yes, that's me," I said. I grabbed my purse, and I got up from my chair as I placed the magazine back on the table. I noticed some people were looking at me strange as I walked toward the door, which I also thought was strange too. *Why did they call my name so soon?* I thought to myself.

"Hi, Dr. Thompson is ready to see you. Can you follow me please?"

DETERMINATION

Hum, that's weird. I thought as I walked through the door. I looked back into the waiting room thinking that there were a lot of people ahead of me. *Why did she call my name before theirs? That's strange,* I thought

"How are you doing today?" she asked.

"I'm fine," I said. And how are you?

"I'm fine, thanks for asking," she said.

"Can you come with me, please?" she asked. I followed her toward the scale that stood against the wall. "I need to weigh you first before you can see Dr. Thompson," she said.

"Oh—okay," I said.

I walked over to the scale, and I put my purse down on the floor. "Can I take off my shoes first?" I asked.

"Sure," she said. Do what you like. I felt a little awkward someone told me that before you step on a scale to take your shoes off first because your shoes added on an additional five pounds.

I took my shoes off as I stepped on the scale. She began to move the balance beams to get my exact weight. She stopped the beam as it pointed at 135. She logged my weight down in my file. "Okay," she said. You can come with me now.

I put my shoes back on as I picked my purse up. I followed her into one of the patient rooms. "Please take a seat," she said. Dr. Thompson will be with you in minute.

"Okay, thanks," I said. I sat down on the examining table as she closed the door, but I got up and walked over to the little round table that stood near the window. There were a lot of magazines on top of the table, so I picked up one of the magazine as I went and sat back down on the examining table while I waited anxiously for Dr. Thompson to arrive.

As I sat reading various articles, I looked up at the clock wondering why it was taking Dr. Thompson so long to come in to see me. An hour had passed, and she still hadn't walked through the door yet. I got up again, and I walked back over to the table to get another magazine to read. I sat back down, but at this time, I was simply thumbing through the magazine because I was getting worried.

My gut feeling was telling me that something wasn't right because there were too many people sitting in the waiting room that was way ahead of me. *So why did they call my name before theirs?* I thought.

While I waited, I thought about the first time I met Dr. Thompson. I had brought my daughter in for her vaccination shots. I was stunned to see a woman doctor for the first time, as I was raised in Alabama where I sort of lived a sheltered life. Plus, I only been living in Dallas for a couple years, and I really hadn't had a reason to go in to see a doctor until then. I was so ignorant back then, thinking all doctors were men, but she proved me wrong. She was so pretty, and she had such a great personality that went with it. I came back to reality, and here I was, still sitting waiting for her to come in to see me.

As I looked at the clock on the wall, I noticed that it had been almost two hours now, and she still hasn't appeared yet. *Where can she be?* I asked. I begin to pace the floor when finally, the door opened, and it was my doctor. "Hi," I said.

"How's it going?" she asked.

"Oh, I'm fine."

"Good."

I went and sat back down on the examining table as I watched her grabbed a small stool that stood against the wall. She sat down and rolled the stool toward me. I gave her my full attention as she open up my folder.

"Your blood work is back from the lab," she said. She took a deep breath. "It looks like you're not an anemic as we first thought. But I do notice that your white blood counts are tremendously high, and they are way above the average limit," she said.

"Okay," I said.

She took another a deep breath. "We think you have Leukemia."

"What!? No! No—Oh God—No!" I screamed. I got up out of my chair and walked around the room pacing the floor. I was so shock over the news that my heart was pounding so hard that I didn't know what to do. "No! No!" I kept screaming. I walked toward the window as I stood there breathing so hard that I couldn't even break a tear because I was hurting so badly inside. "Oh—God!" I said.

I stood looking out the window watching the traffic on Beltline Road as the cars was passing by, but I could hear her talking to me though I was so hurt that I was unable to understand what she was trying to tell me. I'd blocked everything and everybody out of my mind because all I could remember were those last few words that she said to me. *"You have Leukemia."*

I stared through the blinds in a daze thinking that my life had came to a complete stop, but as I stood there, I tried to convince myself that this happened to me for a reason, and it wasn't my place to question God. I just needed to wait this out and see what was in store for me, but I was hurting inside and still couldn't catch my breath.

The tear wouldn't fall from my eyes as I stood looking out the window. I guess reality hadn't kicked in yet that I had a fight on my hands. "People are living longer lives with this disease. I've just got off the phone with this wonderful doctor who specializes in blood diseases at the Medical Center of Plano. I'm going to have one of my nurses drive you to the hospital where he's waiting for you. Okay?" she said.

As I took a deep breath the tears begin to fall, but I just couldn't stop weeping and breathing so hard over the shock because I was so afraid of the unknown and what I was about to go through when I got to the hospital. "Everything is going to be okay," she said. "My nurse will be in with you in a minute, okay?"

"Okay," I said.

I couldn't sit down. I just stood there staring out the window. *"Not me, I can't be sick." I just can't,"* I kept saying to myself.

The door opened. "Ms. Robinson?" I turned around looking at the door. "Hi, I'm here to drive you to the Medical Center of Plano," she said. Are you ready? I took a deep breath and I nodded my head. Grabbing my purse, I walked out the room and followed her into the hallway. I tried to catch my breath, but it got to the point that I couldn't stop. It was if my body took over.

Once we walked into the hallway, I followed her toward the opposite side of the hallway where we exit outside into the parking lot. As we passed my car going toward her truck, I thought, *Will I ever get my life back? Will I be able to do the things that I use to do? What about my daughter?*

She had just made it home after spending her summer with her grandparents in Florida. *How am I going to break the news to her that her mom is very sick? Who's going to pick her up from school? What's my boyfriend going to think once I break the news to him that I have Leukemia?*

She turned off the alarm, and I heard the doors clicked open. I walked to the passenger side and opened the door, got in, and sat down. Once she sat down on the driver side, she started the car and began to back out of her parking space, but I was unable to look over at her. I was a total mess as I put my seat belt on.

I stared outside the passenger window as she made a right turn onto Preston Road. I was so afraid—I didn't know what to expect when once I got to the hospital. All my life I had feared hospitals, but now I had to learn how to face my fears *for the first time.*

On this particular day, it was very hot and sunny especially during the month of August, and the weather was always above one hundred degrees during that time of year. It had to be at least five o'clock in the evening because the traffic was beginning to pick up as the cars were passing us going at least fifty to sixty miles per hour

Determination

in a forty-five mile per hour zone. Now, I would be one of them rushing to get to reach my own destination.

She stopped at the traffic light on Arapaho Road and I glanced out the window as I tried to remember everything that I saw that day. There was a very large and beautiful tree that stood right at the corner of the street. I looked up at the dark green leaves that were blowing in the hot summer air. The sky was blue and very clear that I could see various forms of white clouds as she proceeds down Preston Road.

Why didn't I notice these things before? I kept asking myself. I was always rushing and so impatience about so many things that I didn't see what was really in front of me, until now. Not until I had to find out that I was very sick. Only then did I begin to appreciate God's creation. I should've stopped a long time ago to enjoy the world around me, but I was always in a hurry for a lot of crazy reasons. But not anymore, I had just been diagnosed with Leukemia, and my life was on the line. It was clear to me as she drove me to the hospital that it was important for me that I made a memory of everything that I saw that day.

I heard her talking to me, but I was in my own world. I knew she was trying to give me encouragement, but I couldn't do anything but sit there and cry. Once she got closer to Frankford Road, she made a sharp right turn. "There are so many people who have Leukemia, and they are living longer lives, and you're going to be fine," she said.

I took a deep breath. Suddenly, I stopped thinking about myself and thought about my daughter because somebody had to pick her up from school. "I need to call my boyfriend at work so that he can pick my daughter up from school," I said.

"We can take care of that for you," she said. As she made a left turn onto Coit Road, my heart begins to beat even harder because I could see the hospital from a distance. I sat up in my seat as I tried to convince myself that this happened to me for a reason. I took in a deep breath. "Oh—God," I said softly.

She looked over at me. "It's going to be okay," she said.

As she crossed the railroad tracks and proceeded down Coit Road, she had to stop at the traffic light at the intersection of Plano Parkway. The hospital was only a block away. The traffic light turned green as she proceeds across Fifteenth Street and made a right turn into the hospital parking lot.

She parked her truck, we got out, and I followed her through the sliding doors of the emergency room as we walked up to the receptionist desk. "Excuse me," she said. Hi, I have Dr. Howard's patient.

"Your name, ma'am," she asked me.

"Um…Deagara Robinson," I said.

"Can you spell your first name for me, please?"

I spelled my first name for her. The receptionist checked her computer for my name. "Yes," she said and directed her attention to the nurse at my side. "She has to see one of the clerks for admissions in one of the open booths on your left. I'll let one of them know that you're here, and they'll call her up for more information then," she said.

I followed the nurse as she showed me where to sit until one of the clerks called my name. "Ms. Robinson, I'm going to leave, but they're going to call you up so that they can admit you into the hospital," she said with a caring expression in her voice.

"Okay, thank you," I said.

"Good Luck."

"Thanks."

I begin to cry as I watched her walked through the sliding doors heading toward the parking lot. I sat there wonder how I was I going to break the news to my mother. Four years ago she had been diagnosed with breast cancer, and now I had to call to tell her that I had Leukemia. *How can I tell her? How?* I kept asking myself. I knew eventually I had to tell her, but I didn't want her to worry about me. I was the only child she thought she didn't have to worry about because I was so independent.

IN DENIAL

I was finally called by one of the clerks. I sat down outside of the booth. "Can I have your last and first names please?" she asked. Reality begins to hit me. "Um—Robinson, Deagara," I said softly.

"Can you spell your first name for me, please?"

"Um—D E A G A R A."

"Do you have insurance?" she asked.

"Yes," I said. I pulled the card out of my purse.

"Is it HMO or PPO?" she asked.

"Um—I don't know," I said. I looked at my insurance card, and I noticed PPO was printed on the far right corner of my insurance card. "It looks like its PPO," I said. I handed the card to her, but I thought, *What's the difference?*

"Can I have your home address, please?" she asked.

As I gave her this information, I was looking around thinking, *What am I getting ready to go through?*

"Do you have a will?" she asked.

"Um—yes. I'm sorry, I mean, no."

"Are you a smoker?"

"No."

"Do you drink?"

I looked at her like, *Why are you asking me these questions?* "No," I said.

She picked the phone up, and she began to dial. She started talking to someone.

"Yes, this is the Admission Office. Dr. Howard patient is here," she said. Can you have someone come down, please? She hangs the phone up.

"Okay, Ms. Robinson, they are bringing someone down to take you up to the fourth floor," she said.

"Can I walk up there by myself?" I asked.

"No," she said. Once you've been admitted into the hospital someone has to take you up as a patient. Can you take a seat over there? They should be down in a minute. Okay?"

"Okay, thanks," I said.

As I waited, a man appeared in front of me with a wheelchair. "Ms. Robinson?" he asked.

"Yes," I said.

"Will you come with me, please?" I got up out of my seat as I looked around trying to see if anyone was looking. I sat down in the wheelchair as he kneeled down and pulled the black rubber leg-rest down so I could rest my feet on them.

"Can you place your feet in the leg-rests for me?" he asked.

"Okay," I said. I placed my feet on the leg-rests.

"Thank you," he said. As he pushed me down this long hallway, I became very cold that I could feel little bumps on my arms as he turns the corner toward the elevators. Once we got close to the elevator, he hit the up button as we waited for the elevator to open. He pulled the wheelchair inside of the elevator and he hit the fourth floor button.

The elevator closed, and we began to go up. I thought about this talk show that I watched on television a couple of months before. The topic was about a mother who was trying to save her dying son, who was diagnosed with Leukemia. She had a difficult time locating a donor. Her last alternative was having another baby to see if the infant was a match to her son. The mother became pregnant, and luckily, her daughter was a match, which saved her son's life.

As the elevator doors open, I noticed a nurse's station on the right side of the hallway. I noticed there was couple of nurses standing behind the counters as one of them instructed him to take me down the hall to a room they had already assigned for me. There was nurses walking in the hallway, and I noticed others in patients' rooms attending to them as he pushed me down the hallway.

Once we entered the room, I saw there was a small dressing room area with a door that he opened with one hand, as he pushed me into a much larger room. As he pushed the wheelchair toward the foot of the bed, I got out of the wheelchair and sat on the edge of the bed. "Ma'am, you can change into this gown that they left for you at the foot of the bed," he said.

I looked over at the gown, but I wasn't ready to remove my clothes until I've spoken to my doctor. "Your doctor should be in to see you soon," he said as if reading my thoughts.

"Okay," I said.

As he walked out the door with the wheelchair, I got up and I begin to pace the floor. I just couldn't sit still. I wanted my doctor to come in to tell me from his or her own mouth that I definitely had Leukemia.

I immediately reached for the phone that was sitting on the nightstand by the bed, and I decided to call my boyfriend, James, at his job. "Hey," I said, trying to act casual.

"Hey, what up?" he asked.

"I'm at the hospital. My doctor just told me that I have Leukemia."

"What?!"

"Yes."

The phone went quiet.

I begin to cry again because earlier we had discussed that I should go in to see a doctor, as he was concerned too.

"Are you sure you have Leukemia?" he asked.

"That's what my doctor told me, but I'm waiting to find out from my new doctor." I said.

"It's going to be okay," he said. Everything is going to be fine, DD. Do you need me to pick Lauren up from school?

"Yes, if you could?" I asked.

"Sure."

"Oh, my car is still at the doctor's office," I said. One of the nurses from the doctor's office took me to the hospital.

"Oh—okay. I'll take care of it for you. Are you going to be okay?" he asked.

"Yes, I guess."

"Well, I'll be there after I picked up Lauren."

"Okay," I said.

We hung up as I sat on the hospital bed, waiting for my doctor to walk into the room. I walked over toward the window, and I looked out toward Fifteenth Street. I thought again about how tired I felt when I tried to get up for work when I had to lay back down as I prayed to God to give me enough strength to get back up.

However, I was still trying to figure out how I was going to break the news to my mom. *How I'm I going to pick up the phone and tell her that I have Leukemia?* I remember the day when she broke the news to me that she had breast cancer. I was so devastated.

I sat on the phone with her crying, as she tried to convince me that she was going to be okay. "Dee, the doctors felt that they caught it in time," she said. Stop crying.

"But—Momma," I said.

"It's going to be okay because I'm going to fight this," she said.

I just didn't like to see my mother suffer because she lived in Alabama, and I was all the way in Texas. I was still trying to figure out what I wanted to do with my own life, and I couldn't afford to take off my job to go home. I was barely making enough money to take care of myself and my child.

There was a knock at the door as I saw a nurse walk in.

"Hi, how are you doing?" she asked.

"I'm fine," I said.

"My name is Jane, and I'm here to take your blood pressure and temperature. Can you come and lie down on the bed for me, please?" she asked.

"Sure," I said.

Once I lay down on the bed with my shoes still on my feet, she asked, "Can you open your mouth for me?" I opened my mouth, and as she put the thermostat under my tongue, she continued her questions, "Can you hold your arm out for me?" I held my arm out as she placed a round black plastic sack around the upper part of my arm and began to squeeze the black pump.

As she looked down at her watch, I begin to feel the air in the sack getting tighter and even tighter around my arm. I barely felt any circulation in my arm as she looked at her watch while she released the pressure from my arm.

The thermostat beeped. "Open, please," she asked. I open my mouth. She looked at the thermostat as she logged it down in my file. She took the bag from around my arm. "A lab technician will be coming in later to take blood samples for testing," she said.

"Okay," I said.

"Am I going to die?" I asked her. I thought to myself, *Like she really knew the answers.* She looked at me with hesitation on her face.

"I don't know, but they think yours in its early stage, but your doctor will be able to answers all your questions and your concerns, Okay?" she said.

As I watched her walk out of the room, I got up from the bed, and again, I started pacing the floor. "I got to call my job," I said. I had been working for three years at a law firm downtown, and I told my manager that I would call her once I knew something.

I really enjoyed my job because there wasn't a day that I didn't learn something new. Plus, I was getting a lot of experiences, too. I also loved a challenge. I called my job, and I spoke to the receptionist. "Hi, can I speak with Susan? This is Deagara," I said.

"Sure, Deagara, please hold," she said.

A couple seconds later Susan answered. "DD, is everything okay?" she asked.

"Susan, I've been admitted into the hospital. My doctor just diagnosed me with Leukemia," I said.

"Oh—DD. Are you going to be okay?" she asked

"I don't know. I'm waiting for my doctor to come in to see me, but I'm not sure when I will be back to work," I said.

The phone went silent for a while. "You get better first DD, and I will notify human resources about your situation," she said. And I'll let everyone else know too, okay?

"Okay," I said.

"You take care of yourself, and you'll hear from us soon. Okay?"

"Okay, thank you, Susan."

Once I hung the phone up, I couldn't put it off any longer. I had to call my mom. I hesitated because I still didn't know how I was going to break the news to her that I have Leukemia. *How?* I kept asking myself. I was her only child that wanted their independence so bad and made the decision to leave Montgomery, Alabama, to move six hundred miles away to Dallas, Texas.

For a long time I relied on myself because I wanted it that way. I knew exactly what I was doing when I left. I had my mind set, and I was determined to do it on my own. I had all these goals and dreams I had for myself and my daughter.

"I better call Momma," I said aloud. I took a deep breath as I dialed home. *How is she going to take the news that I have Leukemia?*

DETERMINATION

I asked myself. The phone rung twice, and then she picked the phone up. "Momma," I said.

"Yea," she said.

"It's me, Dee." I start crying again.

"What's wrong?"

"I've been admitted into the hospital, Momma."

"What!?"

"I have Leukemia," I said.

"What...Dee?!" The phone went silent.

"Momma I'm so sacred."

"It's going to be okay. Oh—Dee. Which hospital are you at?" she asked.

"Um—I'm at the Medical Center of Plano," I said.

"I'll be there soon. Okay?"

"Okay, Momma," I said.

I took a sigh of relief because she was willing to come to be with me, but I felt my mother's pain when I broke the news to her. I didn't want to put this on her because she already gone through enough. "I'm coming to Dallas," she said. "Where's Lauren?"

"She's at school, but James going to go pick her up," I said.

"Okay." She took a deep breath. "Oh my goodness," she said very calmly. We're going to make it, Dee. Everything is going to be all right, and somehow, I'll get there. Okay?

"Okay," I said.

"Did you tell Mrs. Scott, yet?"

"No. Not yet. But I'm about to call her right now because someone need to watch Lauren until I get better," I said. She was silent.

"Well, okay. Let me figure out how I'm going to get there. Okay?"

"Okay," I said.

After I got off the phone with my mother, I decided to call Mrs. Scott, my daughter's paternal grandmother. She's a registered nurse, so I figured she would probably know more about this disease and probably could explained it to me much better because I didn't have a clue.

"Hello? Mrs. Scott?"

"Yes," she said.

"This is Dee."

"Hey, Dee, how you're doing? Is everything okay?"

"No, I'm in the hospital right now, Mrs. Scott," I said.

"Yes?"

"They just diagnose me with Leukemia."

"Oh my goodness, Dee," she said. Are you okay?

"I don't know too much right now; I'm still waiting for my doctor to come in to see me."

"Oh, okay."

"Mrs. Scott, I might need you to watch Lauren until I get better," I said.

"Sure. I'll get on the phone right now with my travel agent to see if she could find me some airline tickets to fly down there as soon as possible. It will probably take me a couple of days before I can get there," she said.

"That's fine, Mrs. Scott, thank you," I said.

"Where's Lauren, right now?" she asked.

"She's still at school, but James is picking her up from school right after he gets off of work."

"Oh…okay. Well, let me do some calling, and I should be there soon, Dee."

"Thank you, Mrs. Scott. I really appreciate this."

"No problem, Dee, that's why we're here," she said.

When I hung the phone up, I thought was it a good idea to let my daughter stay with her until I got out of the hospital? Lauren just made it back home two weeks ago after spending the summer with them, but I thought it was too late to change my mind. It's done.

The door open, and it was a lab technician. She had a large tray in her hand with a lot of plastic clear tubes with various colorful lids on top. "Hi, I'm here to draw some of your blood for testing," she said. I looked at her with shock on my face.

"Why?" I asked.

She smiled. "The lab needs to test your blood so that your doctor can have an accurate diagnosis. Can you lie on the bed for me, please?" she asked.

I lay back on the bed. She asked me which arm she could use. I looked at her with hesitation in my face. "I don't care. I guess the left one," I said. As she wrapped a thick rubber cord around my arm, I turned my head the opposite way so that I couldn't see her stick the needle in my arm.

I felt her rubbing something wet on my arm, which I noticed by the smell was rubbing alcohol. She began to move my arm around so that she could locate a good vein. Eventually, I felt a little sting. I lay there with my head turned the opposite way, but I noticed that it was taking her a while so I turned around. It was then that I realized that she had to fill all of the tubes on her tray.

She took the needle out my arm and placed a band-aid there. "Dr. Howard should be in to see you soon okay," she said.

"Thanks," I said.

I got up again, walked over, and sat down in the chair by the window. I thought about how my muscles were always sore for a week after I exercised or lifting weights because it normally took two to three days before the soreness went away, but I felt then that something wasn't right. I never once thought it would be as dramatic as Leukemia.

After some time, there was a knock at the door. As I looked up, I noticed a very tall slim and attractive young white man came in with a file in his hand. He wore a white linen jacket with his nametag pinned on the pocket of his jacket. "Ms. Robinson?" he asked.

"Yes," I said.

"Hi, my name is Dr. Howard," he said. I'm your oncologist. We shook hands.

"Dr. Thompson recommended me," he said. How are you doing?

"I don't know," I said. Is it true? Can there be a mistake?

"There's no mistake, Ms. Robinson. You have Leukemia. You have AML, and we need to start treatment immediately."

I sat back down in the chair, and I put my hands over my faces. "Oh—God," I said. This time the tears fell from my eyes without any hesitation.

"Do you have any questions?" he asked.

"Am I going to live?" I asked.

"There are people who are living with Leukemia, but we won't know that until we do more tests and start you on chemotherapy. We have to put you in remission first, and then we can discuss your options. First, I need you to get undress, and one of the nurses will come in to see you in a few minutes. Okay?" he said.

I held my head down with so much frustration. I didn't know what to think. All I knew was that I had cancer, and I had a battle ahead of me. I took a deep breath and shut everything around me out. I just sat there. I don't even remember when the doctor left the room.

I pulled myself together; I got up, walked toward the bed, to changed my clothes as instructed. *Is this really happening to me? Not me.* I thought. I wanted so—bad to say, *Why me God?* I was too afraid. I was taught not to ever question God. I was scared but still in denial.

James and Lauren walked into the room. James came toward me and gave me a hug while I cried on his shoulder. "It's going to be okay DD," he said. As we pulled away, I nodded my head.

"I know."

"Has the doctor come in yet?"

"Yea," I said.

"What did he say?"

"He said that I have Leukemia."

"Okay," James said. He sat as we talked for a while, but soon, I told him that it was best that he took Lauren home so that she could eat dinner and get ready for school for the next day.

I finally got undress, and I put on the gown that was still lying at the foot of the bed. I laid there under the covers for a while as I watched television. A woman entered the room.

"Hi, how you doing?" she asked. My name is Sharon, and I will be helping Dr. Howard with the bone biopsy procedure.

"The—what?" I asked.

"We need to check your bone marrow so that we can determine how far your prognoses are. However, first you need to take these two pills so that it can relax you before the procedures," she said.

"Oh—okay," I said.

It was only then that I noticed she had two capsules in a small paper cup. She reached out her hands to place them in the palm of my hand. I put the pills in my mouth, as she reached over to the nightstand and gave me the large container of water to swallow them down.

"Thanks," I said. She smiled. I swallowed the pills down, and I gave her the container.

"Just relax and the doctor will be in soon," she said.

"Okay."

As I laid there watching television, I eventually became very sleepy, but as I woke up, I was moaning and unable to move. I felt a sharp pain in my lower back. I closed my eyes so tight. I wanted the pain to stop. Suddenly, I felt someone holding my hand. I squeezed even tighter as the pain increased.

"I'm here, hold on," she said. You're doing fine. I recognized the voice. It was the same nurse who put those pills in my hand. I began to moan even more, but I wouldn't open my eyes because I could feel the tip of the needle as it entered my back again. "It's going to be okay. We're finished," she said.

The tears start rolling down my face. Once I open my eyes, I saw her pretty face smiling back at me, but I was so out of it that I just laid there in that one spot, too afraid to move a muscle. I eventually went back to sleep.

Later on that evening, the door open, and this time there was a very tall black man who came into the room pushing a wheelchair.

"How you're doing?" he asked.

"I'm fine," I said.

"I'm here to take you downstairs for X-rays."

"Oh, okay," I said. None of it was clicking yet. At that point, I was willing to do whatever they asked of me—if it was going to make me better.

I got up. As I held onto the back of my gown with one hand, I walked toward the wheelchair to sit down. As my bareback touched the seat, I became very cold, which brought a chill throughout my body. He kneeled down to make sure my feet were in the leg-rest, and he wrapped a blanket over my lap.

He pushed me down the hallway toward the elevator. I begin to cry because I felt something wasn't right as he pressed the down button. The doors opened. As he pushed the wheelchair inside of the elevator, he pressed the first floor button. Once the elevator doors open to the first floor, I became scared that I begin to shiver as I cried at the same time.

He pushed the wheelchair out of the elevator. I was so cold. When I looked down at my feet, I realized that I didn't have any shoes on. I suddenly realized that I went down the elevator barefooted. There was a hallway that stood slightly toward the left once we got off the elevator. As we entered the hallway, he opened the first door on the left.

By this time, I was shivering like a scared puppy. With one hand, he pushed the wheelchair into this large room. I noticed a very long and large silver table with a lot of white sheets on top of it and a lot of light fixtures that hung from the ceiling above the table. There were two people with blue scrubs on with masks hanging across their necks while they talked among themselves.

He pushed the wheelchair toward the opposite side of the room. There was a large object hanging from the wall. "Can you stand up for me please?" he asked.

I got up, and I walked up toward the wall where the X-ray machine was hanging. He asked me to stand in various position as I held my breath each time, but I just couldn't stop crying and shivering because I was so cold.

"You can sit back down in the wheelchair," he said. I picked up the blanket that I had laid in the chair, and I sat back down in the wheelchair.

I covered my whole body up with the blanket. "I'll be back in a second," he said. I sat there looking around shivering and crying at the same time as I watched the two men who were standing by the table talking as they were preparing for some type of procedure.

I noticed they were playing rock music while they talked among themselves as if I wasn't even there. I sat there just looking at them wondering when the nurse would be coming back to take me back to my room or what was next they would be asking of me? The guy came back into the room, and he pushed the wheelchair toward the long table where the two men were standing.

I looked back at him as he reached down to pull the leg-rest from under my feet. I held my feet up but I was still looking at him with a look of confusion on my face.

"I need you to lay down on the table for me please," he said. I began to cry even more as I looked around at the two men. I put my feet on the cold floor as I got on top of the table. I gradually sat down, but I didn't have a clue what was about to happen.

"Can you bring your body down the table just a little?" one of them asked me. I gradually moved down the table. "That's fine, right there," he said.

As I lay down and turned my head toward one of them, he looked at me because he wanted my full attention. "Hi, my name is Brad. I'm an Anesthesiologist," he said. "I'm going to give you something that's going to relax you and put you to sleep throughout the surgery. Okay?"

"Okay," I cried.

As I watched him rubbed the alcohol on my arm, I realized he was having a difficult time finding a good vein in my arm. I turned my head because I just didn't want to watch him poke me various times. My arm was already black and blue from them previously drawing blood various times in that same arm.

He tried to locate a good vein in my arm, but he was still having a very difficult time. (*I guess because my skin being dark.*) He moved my arm from side to side into the light but still nothing. Eventually, he had no choices but to put the needle on the back of my hand.

He placed a lot tape around the needle so that it wouldn't come loose. He connected the IV onto the needle as I watched him insert the syringe into one of the cords. He turned and smile at me. "Ms. Robinson, I want you to count backward starting from ten," Brad said. Can you do that for me please?

They turned the music up louder, and I counted backward. But before I could get to five, I was out. Something strange happen I woke up; I notice that the music wasn't playing anymore. I could hear voices talking over me. I was too afraid to move. I noticed my head was tilted to the side. I tried to remember what had just occurred. It came back to me that I was still in surgery.

I notice that the music wasn't playing anymore. I could hear voices talking over me.

"What happen to the music?" I asked. I could hear a grasp in the room. There was a pause for a second, and they went completely silent.

I turned my head when I noticed I was covered with white sheets.

"Ms. Robinson?" someone asked.

"Yes," I said.

"We're almost finished. Okay?"

I felt a sharp pain around my upper right side of my chest as the surgeon began to put pressure against it. "Hold on. There's going to be a little pulling, okay?" the surgeon said.

"Okay," I said.

I lay with my eye shut praying to God to give me strength. I was still numb during the entire process. I eventually went back to sleep. I woke up later on in the same hospital room, but I was so drowsy that I laid there wondering if all of this was a bad dream. But it wasn't. It was all true. I turned around to my side slowly, and I looked up and there was an IV attached to a clear bag that was next to the bed. There were various tubes that were running from my chest.

I could actually feel a very small and hard device on the right side of my chest, but I was too afraid to look at it. I laid there crying. *Just try not to lose your faith, DD*, I said to myself. *God didn't give you something that you couldn't handle.*

I tried to sit up, but I was too sore. So I laid there feeling that my body had been invaded.

I eventually pulled myself up slowly. I look over and realize that my doctor must have started me on chemotherapy because there was actually two bags attached to the pole, and I could see two tubes that was attached to my chest. I heard the devices; it sounded like a little motor that was inside of my chest, but I was so tired from the anesthetic that I went back to sleep.

Days had passed before I realized that they had already moved me into another room. I was told by one of the nurses that they usually put all cancer patients in a room by themselves because they didn't want them to get an infection while their immune system was so low due to their chemotherapy treatment.

As I lay in my bed, I saw there was a thirteen-inch television mounted up against the wall diagonally in front of me. I slowly turned to watch television about some breaking news of a major car accident that happened in Europe. I turned up the volume with the remote control so that I could hear clearly what was said, but they wouldn't say who the person was.

It had to be someone very important because they showed a lot of coverage on mostly all the television stations. I was still puzzled because I wanted to know who they were talking about. I was still a little drowsy from the medication, but I slowly turned my body around to the side so that I could have a better view of the television so that I could find out who this person was.

They eventually announced her name. *No—*, I said to myself. I gradually sat up in bed. *Is she okay? What happen?* I kept asking myself. But as I watched the footage from the accident, they finally pronounced that she had passed away. I always thought she was a beautiful woman. I often saw her in most of the tabloids whenever I was waiting in line at the grocery stores though I never picked up one to read about her because I thought it was all gossip anyway.

For several days, I watched all the footage of her life and how she was loved around the world. As I watched the major networks, they spoke so highly of her that I fell in love with her too. She was realistic, and it was unfortunate that she was taken away so tragically.

After each treatment, a nurse came in fully covered with a mask on with long gloves that was all the way up close to her armpits. She carried the chemo in medium size plastic container with a sign that said: *Hazard.* I laid there looking at her as she replaced the bag on the pole and connected the IV to my implanted port. I watched it drip into my veins.

Every four hours, the medical assistants came into my room to check my temperature and blood pressure or to change the sheets on the bed. Later on that day, the dietician provided me with a list of menus to choose what meals I wanted while I was in the hospital. If it was late at night and I wanted a snack, they kept Jell-o or Popsicles on the fourth floor in the nurse's break room.

I met various people who worked at the hospital that came into my room for various reasons. Some were willing to share their stories about their struggle with cancer and how they survived. A lab technician came into my room for blood work, and she told me that she was diagnosed with cancer seven years before. One lady came in to mop the floor, and she told me she had breast cancer five years before, and she was doing fine.

I was getting encouragement from total strangers, who were willing to share their experiences with cancer and how they were willing and determine to fight. I stopped feeling sorry for myself as I realized that I had a chance to change this whole ordeal. I wasn't promise tomorrow even if I wasn't sick. I was stricken with Leukemia, and I knew it wasn't up to me, and I needed to learn how to put a lot of my faith in God.

My doctor visited me every day to check on me and to see if I had any questions. He explained some of the long-term effects of my treatment including the early stage of Menopause. I was thirty-two years old at the time and that word was very foreign to me.

As I laid there watching television, I heard the door open. "Dee?" I looked up toward the door. It was Mrs. Scott.

"Hey, I got here as fast as I could," she said. Are you okay?

"Yes, I'm fine," I said.

"What's the doctor saying?"

"He's doing more tests, but I have Leukemia. He's trying to put me in remission for now."

She took a sigh of relief as she sat down in the chair next to my bed. "Where's Lauren?" she asked.

"She's at school. James should be picking her up from school right about now. So, they should be here pretty soon," I said.

I could tell that Mrs. Scott was exhausted from her flight. "Have you heard from your mother yet?" she asked.

"Yes, I have. She'll be coming down soon."

"Good."

"How was your flight?" I asked.

"It was good," she said.

The door open, and it was Lauren and James. Lauren ran over to her grandmother and gave her a hug.

"Mrs. Scott, this is my boyfriend, James. James this is Lauren's grandmother, Mrs. Scott," I said.

"Hi, how you doing?" he asked

"Fine," she said.

James gave me my keys to my car. "Your car is at home," he said. I picked it up from the doctor's office.

"Oh, okay," I said. Thank you for doing that for me.

"I took your car to the car wash, too," he said.

"Really, well that was nice of you," I said.

"Oh, here." He hand me a receipt.

"What's this?" I asked.

"That's how much it cost me to get your car washed?"

"Huh?" I asked him.

"You can write me out a check later," he said.

I looked at the receipt. My mouth flew open as I looked down at the receipt. "You actually paid someone to wash my car for $62.00?" I asked him.

"Yea," he said.

"But I never paid this much to get my car wash?"

"It needed to be washed," he said.

"You've got to be kidding me, right?" I asked. But, James, my car never has been so dirty enough that I would pay this huge amount.

I took a deep breath because I knew I didn't need to get upset with him, and I also didn't want Mrs. Scott to see us get into an argument either. *I am in the hospital, not sure if I would ever have the chances to even drive my car again and he goes out and has my car wash without even asking me? What was he thinking?* I thought.

As he sat across the room, he smiled at me, but I thought, *How dumb can you get?* "I'll write you a check later," I said. "But could you take Mrs. Scott to our apartment so that she could get some rest?" I asked.

"Yea, sure," he said.

Mrs. Scott got up and gave me a hug. "I'll be back, Dee."

"Okay," I said. Lauren followed behind her not paying too much attention to me. "Okay…bye, Lauren," I said sarcastically. She smiled at me as she waved good-bye.

I smiled at her because I knew she really didn't understand what was going on, but I was disappointed that I didn't get a chance to put in that quality time with her.

The following day, I had more chemotherapy, and as usual, the nurse came in fully covered. I thought, *If it's that toxic then why are they putting it through my veins? What type of side effect will I have after my treatment? When will my hair start falling out?* It hadn't happen yet, so hopefully it wouldn't.

Everyday, I gargled with medicated mouthwash so that I wouldn't get sores in my mouth from the side effects of chemotherapy. Whenever I had to shower, I had to be extra careful not to get any water in the Catheter that was in my chests because it might cause damage to the implanted port.

But there were other major problems that I worried about. The nurses were constantly changing my bed sheets because I was vomiting or bleeding so badly during my menstrual. Mrs. Scott was nice enough to help me through that difficult time even though I was so embarrassed. They gave me strict instructions not to use razor to shave my armpits or legs because if I accidentally cut myself I might bleed to death since my platelets were so low due to the treatment.

Mrs. Scott went out her way to purchase me an electrical razor. She came to the hospital every morning after she dropped Lauren off at school. She sat with me during the day until it was time to pick Lauren up from school, but I thought, *How long she can be able to stay with us? She has her own family to think about too.*

My conscious bothered me because I was having doubts about letting Lauren go back to Florida. She took good care of her in the past, but my mother hadn't made it yet. I was torn about letting her go because I knew my mother would be very disappointed in me if Lauren wasn't here when she came. I had my differences with Mrs. Scott in the past when it came to my daughter, but I really appreciated that she was here for us though I still felt that I had to protect Lauren from what I was about to go through.

While I lay in bed, I built up enough courage to look down inside of my gown to take a peek at the small devices that they placed inside of my chest. There was clear adhesive tape around the Catheter, but I saw the two pointed devices that they were using to connect the IVs to. I also noticed clear liquid was coming through the adhesive tape.

"Mrs. Scott, should this Catheter be leaking?" I asked.

"No. Why?" she asked.

"I think the fluid is coming out."

Mrs. Scott got up and she looked. "I think you better call the nurse in here." I press the button for the nurse.

"Yes?" she said.

"I think something is wrong. Should this be leaking like this?"

I asked. Before I knew it, I was back in surgery again. I woke up during surgery again because I felt pain in my chest.

"Are you almost finished?" I asked.

The room went silent again. The surgeon looked under the sheets. "Just give me one minute and we'll be finish," he said. After the surgery was done and they took me back to my room, the surgeon stuck his head in my room because he wanted to meet the patient who woke up in the middle of his surgery. I smiled at him, but I went back to sleep because I was so drugged up from the anesthetic.

Once I woke up, I could hear someone whispering. "Come on, Lauren. We need to leave right now. Our plane is leaving soon," she whispered. I open my eyes and I saw my daughter and Mrs. Scott slowly sneaking out of the door. I held my head up.

"What's going on?" I demanded to know. Mrs. Scott turned around quickly because she was shock that I was awake. "We need to leave so we won't miss our flight back to Florida," she said.

"You couldn't say good-bye first?" I asked.

"We didn't want to wake you up," she said.

I looked at Lauren. "Come and give your mom a hug before you leave." She walked toward me, and she gave me a hug.

"I love you," I said.

"I love you too," she said.

"You take care, okay?"

"Okay."

"I'll see you soon."

As I watched my daughter walked out the door with Mrs. Scott, I laid my head back down on the pillow. Tears ran down my face. I wondered would I ever see my baby again. Or did I make the biggest mistake of my life letting my child go back down to Florida?

I knew in the past that Mrs. Scott could be very manipulative. *But could I trust her now while I'm sick? Maybe I'm jumping to conclusions because she did stay around for a while to help me while I was in the hospital, but I need to get better first because I had a fight on my hands. But did I do the right thing by sheltering Lauren from what I'm about to go through? Or should I've let her stay here in Texas with me so that she could understand how cancer affects your life?* Time would tell.

MY BATTLE TO LIVE

After they surgically removed the catheter from my chest, I was very sore and swollen. A nurse came in periodically to change the bandages, which was a very tiresome responsibility for them I'm sure. Because the scar was very tender, I consistently lay wishing that the nurses wouldn't come in to change my bandages.

One nurse came in one morning to change my bandages, but as she pulled the badge off quickly, it felt like she peeled my skin from my body. I yelled so loud that everyone on the fourth floor heard my voice. Some of the nurses ran into my room, trying to figure out what had happen. I don't think she was thinking or she just really didn't know how swollen I was, but she was very apologetic as I lie there crying.

After my doctor visited that morning, I heard him outside my door talking with one of the top oncologist. He was explaining my prognoses and my status to him, and I heard him tell the doctor that I needed a bone marrow transplant to prolong my life. As I lay back in my bed thinking to myself, *How sick am I really? What is a bone marrow transplant? Could I actually die?*

Later on that afternoon, I heard a familiar voice call out to me. "Dee?" I turned my head to the door. "Mama?"

"How you're doing?" she asked.

"I'm fine, I said."

"I got here as fast as I could," she said. I had to take the bus to get here from Montgomery.

"How did you get to the hospital?"

I asked a stranger to give me a ride to the hospital.

"Mama…a stranger," I said.

"Yea, but he was a very nice man though," she said.

She looked around and took a seat next to my bed. I could tell she was exhausted because I saw a sigh of relief on her face that she made it there safely.

"Where's Lauren?" she asked.

"Mrs. Scott took her back to Florida," I said.

"Oh." I saw that she was disappointed.

"Mama, I didn't want Lauren to see me this way considering what I was about to go through."

"Dee, I tried to get here before Mrs. Scott did. Lauren needs to see what it's like to have cancer. You shouldn't try to protect her from this. She needs to see and understand what is going on, Dee," she said.

She sat quietly for a while as she laid back in the chair. "Are you okay?" she asked.

"Yes, but my doctor isn't saying too much though. I don't understand why he's so quiet." I said.

"Well, maybe he'll talk with me then," she said.

"My doctor set up an appointment for me to meet with this physician that specializes in bone marrow transplants," I said.

"You need a bone marrow transplant?" she asked.

"I guess. I don't know," I said.

She took a deep breath. "Okay," she said. Well we'll find out when I see your doctor.

I looked over at my mother she was so exhausted. "Momma, I know you are probably tired, I'll have James come up here after work to pick you up so that you can get some rest." I said.

"Okay," she said.

I called James at his job to see if he could pick my mother up from the hospital and take her back to our apartment so that she could get some rest. Though he said he would, I could tell from his words that we had become distance. We weren't talking as much to one another since I had been diagnosed with Leukemia. He barely came to see me during my treatment. That moral support that I thought would be there wasn't.

I was amazed a couple of weeks ago, we were so close. We talked a lot about our goals and dreams for one another. Strange how quickly things change when I became ill. It was obvious I should've listened to my conscious when I first met him.

I remembered the first time we met. I was at this bar on Greenville Avenue with one of my friends. We stopped for drinks before we headed to the First Friday's Party that was held every month. As we left the bar, James came behind us in the parking lot, and he asked me for my phone number.

I gave him my number, but I didn't think much about him. I'd been stopped a lot by guys who wanted my phone number. At the time, I hadn't found the right man, so I decided to keep giving out my number until the right guy appealed to me.

Once I gave him my number, my girlfriend and I walked to my car. "What you thought about him?" she asked.

"He's nice." I said.

"DD, your standards are too high," she said.

"What?"

"Your standards are too high."

"Because I wasn't excited about this guy, you think my standards are high?" I asked.

"Yea," she said. You need to give someone a chance.

"I don't know," I said. I left the conversation alone that night because I didn't know what I wanted or expected from a man, but

I knew I wasn't going to settle for anybody. Even though things weren't good at the end between my first love, Raymond and I he showed me how a woman should be treated by a man, and I wasn't going to settle for anything less than that!

But what she said to me that night stayed in my head, and I thought that maybe she was right. I thought, *I should give someone a chance.* But I felt that I only had one life, and I wasn't going to date or get involved with anyone whose morals and goals were not set for him. *Goals are important.* I had goals, even though I didn't know which direction I wanted to go when it came to my career.

The first time I spoke with James on the phone, I accidentally got him mixed up with another guy. I was so embarrassed that I hung the phone up. He called me right back. Soon, we started seeing a lot of each other on a regular basis. Once the relationship became serious, he wanted me to change my phone number, due to the large volume of phone calls I was receiving from other men.

I basically had more men friends than women. When I was younger, my mother told me that your best friend is a man just as long you don't sleep with him. You tell a man something private quicker than you can tell a woman because men aren't as fast to gossip. But after a while, I changed my phone number. Three months into our relationship, I pressured him into moving in with me though at first he hesitated. He felt that it wasn't right in God's eyes that we lived in sin.

I couldn't see that at first because I wanted to be in a committed relationship. Eventually, he thought it was a good idea because we could both save money. His family and one of his friends weren't too excited about us moving in together because his mother wanted to move to Texas from Louisiana. She wanted them to be a family again, so she suggested that they get an apartment together. They also thought he should be with a woman who was more passive. *Passive,* I thought. *I don't think that is me. I have been independent all my life, and I learned to solely rely on myself—and God.*

DETERMINATION

Right after we moved in together, I traveled with him to Shreveport, Louisiana, because he was worried about his mother's health and where she was living. He was also concerned that his family was tired of taking care of her. She had nowhere to go and basically noone to rely on but him, so she moved to the country with her aunt. But what I couldn't understand was that she had a home. *Why she wasn't staying in the house?* But he kept saying that she wasn't capable to take care of herself so she lived with family, they were planning on selling her house and putting her in an institution.

Once we arrived in Shreveport, we drove another fifteen minutes to the country to his aunt's house. As we drove down this very narrow two-lane road, I noticed a very small yellow house that stood by itself. He turned onto this property and parked my car in the yard.

We got out as his mother walked out the house to greet us and lead us to the house. As we entered into his aunt's house, I introduced myself to his aunt. We stood in her kitchen for a while, while James talked to his mother.

"Would you like something to eat?" His aunt asked me. We don't have much as you probably have but we get by.

Huh? I thought. *What was that?* I stood there as I watched the expressions on her face, and I realized that she thought I was a snob. I couldn't understand why. *She just met me.* I guessed it came from James' mother though I had showed her a lot of respect when she came to Dallas to visit her son that past summer.

"No, Ma'am," I said. But thank you though.

While James talked with his mother, I sat there trying to figure out why she made such a strong accusation without even knowing me. *Did I give her that impression when I introduced myself that I thought I was better than she was?*

We stayed for an hour as James' mother begged him to let her move to Dallas with him. He held fast to his original decision because he wasn't ready for that responsibility and he needed to get himself together first.

As we walked to my car, she started to cry. "Please let me move to Dallas with you, James. I don't have anywhere else to go. My family doesn't want to have anything to do with me, James," she begged. I stood there with tears in my eyes as she begged her son, but he kept telling her no.

"Not right now, Momma," he said.

"Please, James."

"Momma, I got to get myself together first." He walked over and he hugged her.

"I'll be back down to see you. Okay," he said. As we got into the car and drove back to Dallas, we were quite.

I felt so sorry for her, and I couldn't understand why he didn't want the responsibility and neither did his family. "Dee, she's not responsible. She did this to herself," James said.

"But this is your mother, James," I said.

"We tried everything and some of my family is tired now. They feel that it's my responsibility to take care of her, but I'm not financially ready," he said. I didn't say anything else because I didn't want to get involved with something that I wasn't clear about.

At the time, I was still living in my old apartment. We decided to move into a larger apartment in August. We moved into a larger apartment, The Preston Trace on Frankford Road that was located a couple of miles from where I lived earlier.

James close friend helped us move our furniture into our new apartment. We were unable to move all of our furniture that day. It was getting too late in the evening. I insisted on getting everything moved but James thought it would be best to wait until tomorrow. I wouldn't hear of it. I wanted everything completed especially my thirty-two inch television that would've been left behind until tomorrow.

Once James and his friend took more furniture to our new

Determination

apartment I stayed behind. I decided to drag my television down three flights of stairs to my car. I was just that determine to get my television into my new apartment. Once I dragged the television down the first flight of the stairs, I realized that it was too late for me to turn around and take the television back up the stairs.

As I struggled to get this large television down the stairs, I felt stupid for pulling and dragging this large television down two flights of stairs. I was out of breath and I was tired too. *"Where did I get all of this determination from?"* I said to myself. Because when I had something set in my mind that I was going to do, I normally did it. Which was very stressful and I brought a lot of this pressure upon myself because I wasn't willing to wait until the next day but it was too late.

Eventually, I got the television down the flights of stairs when James and his friend walked up. James looked at me and shook his head. They grabbed the television and they put it in the truck. But boy did I feel stupid that day but once we were settled into our new apartment it came out looking very nice.

We threw my bed away and we used James' bed instead because his bed was much nicer and firmer then the one I had for years But, I begin to noticed that he didn't contributed anything other than his bed and a clock into to our new apartment so it felt like it wasn't ours together.

I brought new paintings and new personal items for the apartment that hung throughout the apartment. Eventually, he brought a computer for his own personal use. I began to think, *Where was he getting the money from? He told me that he was having hard times and that was one of the reasons why he moved in with his friend in Rowlett before we moved in together.*

A couple of weeks after we moved into the apartment, I begin to have flu like symptoms, which I thought was strange because it was August. I was weak and I didn't have any energy. I didn't feel my normal self. I took a couple of days off of work hoping that with a lot of rest I would feel better, but I simply lay in bed, eating soup and drinking orange juice. James slept on the couch in the living room.

He didn't even try to comfort me in anyway by fixing me soup or getting over the counter medication. He did nothing, but I had a good friend, Robert who used to go out his way by calling or stopping by unannounced to make sure Lauren and I were okay.

When I was living alone if I told Robert I had a cold an hour later, he came over. He went to the grocery store and brought me orange juice, soup, and over the counter medication. As I lay in James' bed sick, I thought then that something wasn't right with our relationship.

Later on that night, I got out of the bed, got on my knees, prayed to God, asking him to show me if this was the right man for me. James slept on that couch until he thought I was better. But I never got better; I was diagnosed with Leukemia.

That evening, James came up to the hospital, picked my mother up, and took her to our apartment so that she could get some rest. The next day, I lay in bed and didn't hear from my mother the entire day. I wondered if she was okay. It was almost noon, and this was her first time being in Texas. *I gave her my keys to my car,* I thought. *Maybe she was lost.*

There was a knock at the door. "Mrs. Robinson?" I looked at the door, and I noticed that it was a doctor I had never met before. He walked up and shook my hand. "Hi, how you are doing?" he asked.

"I'm fine," I said.

"I'm Dr. Blake," he said. He was at least six feet tall, slim, and very clean cut. He was also wearing a long linen jacket, but I could tell from his nametag that he wasn't a doctor from the Medical Center of Plano.

"I'll be performing your bone marrow transplant, and I'm here to explain the procedures and what to expect," he said.

DETERMINATION

My what? I asked myself I looked at him puzzled. *My doctor didn't mention to me that I needed a bone marrow transplant...or did he because I only heard him once outside my door talking with the head oncologist, but he didn't actually tell me himself.*

I still didn't understand my prognoses or the medical terminology. It was all foreign to me. It seemed like everything was happening so fast, but all I knew is that I wanted to get better. So, I sat back in the bed, and I listen to every word he had to say so I could ask my doctor when he came to see me later that day.

I noticed that he had a pad in his hand when he walked over by the window and grabbed a chair. He sat down in the middle of the room and crossed his legs. He talked nonstop about the procedure, but I was still unable to understand any of the medical terminology.

As he talked on, I began to understand some of what he was saying to me though still not knowing the first thing I should ask him. I guess Dr. Howard felt that it would be too overwhelming for me because of the way I acted after finding out that I had Leukemia. I guess he probably wanted to wait to discuss this with me until I was rational enough to accept reality.

While I listen to the doctor, he gave me a brief understanding of his position and how he was one of the top bone marrow transplant specialists in the state of Texas. "There is not as many African Americans registered as donors on the National Bone Marrow Registry. So, I feel that it wouldn't be a good idea to put you on the registry," he said. He got my full attention. Everything was clicking in my head. I waited for him to ask me if I had any questions because I wanted to make sure I heard him right.

Wait a minute! I thought. *Didn't he just say he wasn't going to put me on the National Bone Marrow Registry because there's not enough African Americans listed?* "I'm sorry, but I'm confused," I said. "Now, why you're not going to put me on the registry, again?" I asked.

"The proteins in African American and Caucasian's blood are

different, and I think that it would be a waste of time to put you on the registry because there's not enough African Americans on the registry."

"Oh," I said. I didn't know that.

"But we'll start testing your siblings and other members of your family to see if we can find someone who is a match to you."

I was very polite and silent, but I was still unable to understand all the medical terminology so I didn't know what to actually ask him. I was confused. But what stuck in my head was when he said that he wasn't going to put me on the National Bone Marrow Registry because there wasn't enough African Americans listed on the system.

He got up from his chair and he put it back against the wall. "Well, it was very nice meeting you," he said.

"It was nice meeting you too," I said. Thank you.

As he walked out the room, I started crying. I was so angry that I sat there for a while thinking and trying to sink in all of what he told me. As I sat up in my bed, I realized that he wasn't giving me any options by not putting me on the registry. *He just sat in here, in this room, and told me that he wasn't going to put me on the National Bone Marrow Registry because he felt there weren't enough African Americans listed.*

I grabbed the plastic containers that sat on the nightstand, and I threw them across the room. I cried even more. One of the nurses ran into the room. "Are you okay?" she asked.

"No." I said.

"What's wrong?"

"This doctor just told me that he wasn't going to put me on the registry because there are not enough African Americans out there."

"Okay. Calm down. We have Dr. Howard come in to see you later on today, and you can discuss this with him then. Okay?"

"Okay." I lay there for hours thinking, *What if they are unable to find me a match with someone in my family? What's next for me? What options do I have? Will I die?* The nurse told me that there was a gentleman across the hallway, and they found his donor in Germany; their DNA matched five out of six. She also told me that his wife was expecting a baby.

I lay back down, and I looked up at the ceiling, wondering what was going on. There were so many questions that were going on in my head, but at the same time I was wondering, *Where is my mother?* I kept calling my apartment trying to figure out if she was there because I still haven't heard from her.

In the back of mind, I felt that she was somewhere shopping. Dallas was a new territory for her, and I knew she was going to venture out and discovery where the major malls were in the city. My mother loved to shop for sales on clothes and items to decorate her house.

My mother had great taste; I followed her path when it came to clothes and furniture. She always told me to stick with the basic colors, not prints or flowers because they fall out of fashion pretty quickly. She taught me that with basic colors I could wear those clothes for seasons to come and still get the same compliments.

My mother actually remodeled her house by joining two bedrooms so that she had more closet spaces. Even that wasn't enough space for her clothes but she knew when her clothes were missing even though she had so many clothes that it was ridiculous. But what was so weird she knew when something was taken out of her closet.

Our next-door neighbor asked to borrow a sweater to wear to a concert. I decided to let her borrow one of my mother's sweaters. It was a dark hunter green wool sweater that I let her borrow which I thought for sure my mother wouldn't miss until she asked everyone in the house have anyone seen her green wool sweater? I didn't say a thing because I knew our neighbor would bring it back to me the next day.

When our neighbor knocked at the front door, I open the door but I noticed she was holding a small green sweater in her hand that was small enough to fit an infant. "What's this?" I asked her.

"Girl, I washed your mama's sweater and I put it in the dryer," she said.

"What sweater!" Not my mom's sweater!" I said.

She held the sweater up where I could see it. My mouth was wide open with shock. All I could do but to think how my mother was going to kill me if she ever found out which she didn't but I learned then to leave her clothes alone.

As I laid there for a while still worried about my mother, so I called my brother in Alabama to see if he heard from her, but he wasn't there. I spoke with his girlfriend.

"Hey, Monica, this is Dee have you heard from Momma?" I asked. She has been gone most of the day, and I haven't heard from her yet. She has my car, and I'm not sure if she's lost or she gotten into an accident.

"Girl, your momma probably at TJ Maxx, Marshalls, or even Ross," she said. She'll come to the hospital when she's finished shopping.

I took a sigh of relief when she told me that. I felt that was what she was doing. I just needed someone else to confirm it. When she finally arrived to the hospital, I was relieved to see that she was okay. "Momma, I was worried about you." I said.

"Why?" she asked.

"I didn't know if you've gotten lost or in an accident."

"Dee, you don't have to worry about me. I can take care of myself."

I saw the expression on her face. I knew its best that I left that conversation alone. My mother sat down as she took a deep breath. She was exhausted from doing all that shopping.

"Where did you go?" I asked.

"I went to T J Maxx and Marshall," she said. I brought me some shoes and this very cute purse. They're down in the car, but I'll bring them up later so you can see them. Are you doing okay?

"Yea, I'm fine," I said. But, Momma, the doctor who's going to perform the bone marrow transplant came in this morning, and he told me that he thought it wouldn't be a good idea to put me on the National Bone Marrow Registry because there wasn't enough minorities on the registry.

"I don't understand," she said. Why would he say that?

"I don't know, but he said that blacks and whites proteins in our blood are different and that it was a waste of time to put me on the list," I said.

"Have your doctor come in to see you yet?" she asked.

"No, not yet," I said.

"Well, then, we'll ask your doctor then."

I was so happy she was here with me because I knew she would find out what I needed to know. My mother sat next to my bed exhausted after shopping most of the day. She sat and watched television with me while we waited for the doctor.

Later on that day, my doctor came in to check on me. As he entered the room, he introduced himself to my mother. It was brought to his attention by one of the nurses that I was very upset after I met with this doctor earlier today. As he sat down, I told him that I had spoken with the doctor who was suppose to do the bone marrow transplant and how he thought that it wouldn't be a good decision to put me on the national registry because it wasn't enough minorities listed. He didn't say anything.

My mother explained to him how a lot of doctors didn't care that much about African Americans. "I was raised in the south, and I had to experience a lot of prejudice most of my life," she said. Our lives aren't that important to some doctors. I've experienced that myself because there wasn't any urgency to get me the treatment I needed once I was diagnose with breast cancer.

Dr. Howard interrupted my mother. "Mrs. Robinson, I'm sorry, but I'm married to an African American woman." I looked over at my mother; she was stunned. She immediately went silent very quickly. He got up from the chair. "I'll check into this and get back with you both, okay?" he said.

"Okay. Thank you," I said.

After my mother made those remarks to Dr. Howard, I was so embarrassed for her and myself. I didn't know if I wanted to face him the next day. I don't think that she realized that times had changed a lot from those days when she grew up.

A couple of days after the embarrassing episode with my doctor, my mother made friends with a patient that was in the next room. She went over and talked with the man and his wife for hours before she eventually came back to my room. My mother could be the most caring and loving person anyone ever met, but she also loved to talk.

My mother came back to my room, and she told me that the patient next door was a black man in his mid-forties. The husband was diagnosed with Leukemia also, and his wife was there by his side giving him moral support. She told me that he could barely talk because he had so many sores in his mouth from the side effects of the chemotherapy.

She also told me that he knew he had Leukemia for a while, but he didn't want to come in for treatment until it gotten really bad. He didn't know how long he had to live. The doctor tried to see if there were other options out there to save his life, but he insisted on going home to fix his wife's car.

My mother suggested that I go over to meet them, but I was too weak from all the chemotherapy that they put in my body. Plus, I didn't want to talk with anyone at the time. I didn't have an appetite and I basically threw up everything I ate all I wanted to do was just lie there in bed to think what path God was leading me.

Most days, my mother sat with me. But one particular day, James decided to come up to the hospital to visit with me after he got off work. Once he walked into the room, he sat on the other side of the room next to a small office desk that stood near the window. He sat there very quietly for a while. I looked over at him, and I noticed he prop his feet up on the desk while my mother and I watched television.

James and my mother started talking among themselves though, at the time, I wasn't paying any attention. "It's so hard to live with Dee," she said. "She can be a very difficult person sometime." I looked at her shocked. *She would start this now?* "What did I do?" I asked. She just shook her head.

I sat there thinking, *I knew this was going to happen.* That's why I had already explained to James earlier not to play into my mother's manipulative games. She could be very convincing. I even told him not to believe everything that she said about me, that he needed to make his own judgments and not take sides.

James sat in the corner very quiet but had a smirk on his face. I remained quiet. I remembered growing up and being reminded how dark my complexion was on a constant basis. I was told that I was crazy, and I would grow up to be a prostitute, an alcoholic like my father. I was going to be fat, and "Ain't any man going to want you." Those remarks have stayed with me, even when I was young enough to understand what she was saying to me.

When I got a little older, I knew I had to leave Montgomery to find my own direction in life. I was determined to prove my mother wrong.

I didn't want to hear her bashing me in front of him, especially not while I was so sick. "You're right; she can be difficult sometimes," James said. He looked back at me with his feet still prompt on the desk.

"You know what, Mrs. Robinson, she had the nerve to get on me for smoking a joint with one of my friends," he said. He leaned back in the chair even further while one of his feet was still prompt on the desk.

"Dee is crazy," she said.

I looked at both of them. *Crazy!* I thought. I was uses to the verbal abuse from her, but as I sat there looking over at him, I was fuming! I had told him not to take sides but to be open minded. I had told him my mother sometimes talked negatively toward me. I dealt with that most of my life. *And for him to sit in this hospital room after just meeting her several days ago! How dare he?*

I sat up in my bed. I couldn't believe what was coming out of his mouth as he tried to justify that I didn't approve of him smoking a joint in front of my child. *He forgot to mention he was smoking this joint around my eight-year-old daughter! After I explained to him that I don't do drugs and I don't allow drugs around my child. So what was he trying to say that I sometime pulled things out of proportion because he chosen to smoke a joint around my child? Hmm—all right.* I thought to myself.

As I lay in the bed, I thought, *that's all she needs! Someone to agree with her so that she can get started in on me.* It took me over six years to go back home to visit my mother when I moved to Texas. *This was one of the reason I had left. My self-esteem was so low because of her.*

I laid there listening to them go back and forth saying little negative things about me. I was so weak from all the medication and the chemotherapy treatment that I didn't have that much strength to go back and forth with them.

I began to cry because I didn't want to fight with them both. *Not now,* I thought. Not *while everything was so confusing to me.* I had an IV that was hooked up to my Hickman line that sat in the middle of my chest. However, it got to the point that I asked myself, *How much are you going to put up with?*

With what little strength I had in me, I gradually sat up, moved to the side of the bed, and slowly put my feet on the cold floor. I reached over and grabbed the long pole, with various bags of fluid attached that stood in between my bed and nightstand.

I slowly start walking toward James while my mother sat in

the chair next to my bed talking. I pulled the pole with one hand and looked at James with anger in my eyes, as he just sat there wondering what was about to happen. When he noticed that I was getting closer, he placed the legs of the chair back down onto the floor.

Once I was close enough, I started swinging my arms, hitting him with the little strength I had in my body. "You have the nerves to justify what you did! I told you not take sides! I told you!" I screamed.

He started putting his arm up to block my hands. "Get Out!" I screamed. Get Out! Now!

"You're crazy!" My mother screamed.

The nurses came rushing into the room. "Okay, you guys, I'm sorry, but you need to leave," she said. She's very sick, and she doesn't need to be upset right now.

As I struggled back to my bed, I thought to myself, *What just happened?* I was so angry and shocked after what had happen. I was in the hospital fighting for my life, and I wasn't sure if I was going to live or die. To hear people, who said that they loved me, say what they really felt, hurt me so bad.

For two days, I laid in the hospital room all alone with the curtains closed. I didn't want to see or speak to anyone. The nurses came in every four hour to take my temperature and blood pressure or clean the badges from the catheter. They were my only visitors.

"Excuse me." One the nurse stuck her head into my room. But your mother wants to know if it was okay for her to come in to see you," she said.

"No," I said. I was still upset with my mother. *How she could do this to me at a time when I really needed her?* I was so scared of the unknown and down on myself. For her to treat me like that was unthinkable.

Several days later, my doctor scheduled me for another bone biopsy. I requested if I could have the same nurse that held my hand the first time, which they allowed. They provided me medication to relax me for the procedure, and though I was sort of out of it, I still felt the tip of the needle entering my lower back.

I lay on my side with my eyes closed tight, moaning desperately as she held my hand tight hoping he will be done soon. The next day, the results from the test came back. The cancer wasn't in remission. The doctor advised me that I had to go through more chemotherapy. But he had to first wait until my red and white blood cell levels was back up to normal so that my immune system would be able to fight off any infections. Until then, he would release me from the hospital. He discussed with me that they would try to put me in remission, which meant they could store my good white cells and give them back to me—if they couldn't locate a donor.

After almost two months in the hospital, my doctor gave me the okay to go home for a while until my immune system build up for more chemotherapy. This would actually be the first time since I was diagnosed with the Leukemia that I had a chance to go home. When I got there, I mostly laid in the bed just thinking and wondering what was next for me. My life was at stand still. I didn't know what to expect and if I was going to live.

RECAPTURING THE PAST

I lay on my back looking up at the ceiling; I felt like someone had violated my body. I just didn't feel like my normal self. There were two tubes hanging from out of my chest. I was so afraid to lay a certain way while I slept because I might accidently pull the Hickman out my chest and probably bleed to death.

Later on that morning, I got out of bed and walked into the bathroom where I looked in the mirror since I've been home. As I stood there, I realized that my hair was beginning to fall out in patches. A couple a months before, my hair was at my shoulders, but now it fell out as soon as I combed my hair.

I cried as I stood there wanting to ask, *Why me?* But I couldn't. I just couldn't question God. I felt that this happened to me for a reason. I tried to convince myself that there was going to be better days and that one day my hair would grow back. I hoped that God would give me a chance to be more appreciative of what he had blessed me with and my surroundings. However, after my incident at the hospital, my mother had shut herself up in my daughter's bedroom, and she wasn't really speaking to me.

She wouldn't even come out of the bedroom for nothing unless she was going to the kitchen or to the bathroom. I knocked on the door to ask if she wanted me to fix her something to eat or if she needed anything. She would only talk to me through the door with a very dry and direct voice.

I realized then that she had already bought food that she kept in the bedroom so that she could avoid saying anything to me. Eventually, I realized nothing was going to pull her out of that room. She was also hurt—when I didn't want to see her after the incident.

I went back into my room and I lay down for a while.

The phone rung, I immediately picked the phone up. It had been so lonely for me since I got back home I wanted to talk to anybody. "Hello," I said.

"Hey, Dee, where's Momma?" It was my brother.

"She's in the other room."

"Can I speak with her?"

"Yea, sure," I said.

I got up and sat on the edge of the bed. "Scott, Momma won't speak to me. She locked herself in Lauren's room and she won't come out," I said.

"Dee, you and Momma need to learn how to get alone," he said. She loves you and I know you love Momma, but you two are *so* much alike. That's one of the reasons why you guy can't get alone.

"But Scott—"

"Dee, when the both of you are apart from one another, you're the best of friends."

I sat there not saying a word. He was right. My brother was turning into an intelligent man. He was realistic like my father. "Let me get her for you."

I knocked on the door. "Momma, Scotty is on the phone. He wants to talk with you," I said. She slightly opened the door and held her hand out not giving me any eye contact. I gave her the phone, and with a dry voice, she told me, "Thank you." Then she shut the door.

What could I say to change things among us? I was so angry with her at that time, but I'm not anymore. It was a very heated confrontation, but I felt that she took sides with James and that it was okay what James said. But after speaking with my brother, I knew he was right. We just didn't get along when we were around each other, but I loved her so much.

I went back to my room, sat down on the bed, and I thought about what my brother said to me. It made so much sense. I remembered when I moved to Dallas, my mother and I were suddenly best of friends. We would talk and tell each other how much we loved each other, but if we were both in the same room, it was very argumentative.

I couldn't understand that until my brother opened my eyes. I didn't have my mother's complexion, but we did look alike—I was shaped like her too. She had a beautiful body and I admired her so much because she didn't look her age. She had passed that on to my siblings and me.

I was so proud to call her my mom because she had given my siblings and me that compassion and moral values that we carried with us until this day.

Later on that day, I knocked on the door again. "Momma, do you want me to fix you something to eat?" I asked

"No," she said. The following day she left without saying goodbye to me. James drove her to the bus station so that she could go back home to Montgomery.

After she left, I knew then that this was a fight that I had to do alone. I had to learn how to put a lot of my faith in God. I knew I couldn't rely on flesh anymore. I had to learn how to rely on God and myself.

While I was home, my days were slow. I thought a lot about my life in general especially my past. I was born in a small town in Marengo county, Demopolis, Alabama. I was a little dark and skinny girl with an oval face. My hair was short and fine like my father's. I use to envy my sisters, whose hair was very long and thick like my mother. There were six of us—my two sisters, one brother, my parents, and myself.

We lived in a small, predominately-black area of the town on a dirt road in a small white three-bedroom house right off of Highway US 80. We could actually see the highway from our backyard. We had an old rounding washing machine that stood on the back porch where my mother uses to wash our clothes. I often watched her placed them through the rollers to remove excessive water from them before she hung them on the clothesline to dry.

Every Saturday morning, I woke up by the loud noise of my father's lawnmower, and I watched him from my bedroom window as he cut the lawn. My father always had on old clothes with old worn out Stacy Adams shoes whenever I watched him pushing his lawnmower up and down his yard.

My father enjoyed being out in his yard cutting the grass or trimming the shrubs. He always kept our grass cut and watered. He had grown four plum trees in his back yard for each one of his children. During the summer, we would go out in the back yard to pick the plums off the ground once they have fallen off the trees.

There were also two large pecan trees that stood on the side of our house. My sisters and I would sometime play under the shade during the hot summer days. But if the season was right, we would pick the pecans off the ground and try to peal the shells from around the hard nuts. We had to look around in the yard to find something hard to crack the pecans so that we could eat what was inside.

During the summer, my father loved to barbecue outside in the backyard. My parents would sometime invite some of our family over for the Fourth of July; we would then have a large outing in our backyard. My sisters and I had a lot of fun running around playing in the front yard with our cousins while the adults sat in the backyard laughing and reminiscing about the past.

During the Christmas season, our family had a tradition. Our father would go out and purchase the freshest seven-foot Christmas tree in Marengo County. My siblings and I would then sit on the floor as we watched our father decorate our Christmas tree so beautifully.

Afterward, we would turn off the lights as we watched with enthusiasm as the colorful lights blinked in the dark. The house always had a fresh smell of the pine tree during the Christmas season.

We woke up on Christmas morning with toys and gifts scattered on the floor around the Christmas tree where a lot of apples, oranges, and nuts were underneath the tree too. We took turns opening Christmas gifts our parents had surprised us with. I felt very fortunate, as I look back now that God had blessed us with both of my parents. Finally, sometime after midnight, we fell asleep from pure exhaustion.

I can't remember not really wanting or needing anything because we were basically a middle class family back in the early seventies, but our parents taught us about togetherness and moral values—especially love and respect for one another. They taught us at an early age how to say our prayers before we went to bed at night. We use to kneel down on the side of our beds to say our prayer out loud as one of our parents stood listening to us to make sure we were saying them correctly.

Even during dinner, we all took turns saying our favorite verse as my father lead us at the head of the table. When my turn came around, I would say one that I had learned after sitting at my grandparent's dining room's table; they had various scriptures of the Ten Commandments hung on their dining room wall.

Every week, my father drove his red Volkswagen Bug thirty miles from Demopolis to Eutaw, Alabama, to his job where he taught music as a band director and a history teacher at the high school. My mother worked at a Russell Mill plant sewing t-shirts in Demopolis.

When I was very young, we had several babysitters within our community, who watched me while my parents were at work. I actually remembered three of them, one of which lived next door to us and another who lived down the road from our house. The other one I didn't care that much for because she tried to make me eat sweet rice, which I didn't like at all.

She used to sit me down in the middle of the kitchen floor facing the back screen door. She would place a bowl of sweet rice with a spool in between my legs to eat. I stubbornly looked outside the screen door as I watched my oldest sister play with other kids in the backyard.

I just sat there for a while watching them playing rather than eating the bowl of sweet rice. I sat there for a long time not willing to budge a lick as she tried her best to make me eat that rice. She kept coming back into the kitchen to see if I was finished, but I never touched the food.

As she lifts the spoon up toward my mouth, I would close my mouth even tighter and turned my head. After a while, she spanked my legs, but I still wouldn't eat her sweet rice and I didn't see that much of her after that day.

Our next-door neighbor uses to watch my sisters and me most of the time. Her name was Bertha James. I guess I was her favorite because she would let me say whatever was on my mind. I used to stand on my parent's front porch with my hands on my hips fussing back with her as she sat on her porch laughing at me. I was young and a very sassy child at the time that was full of mouth but no action.

During the summer Mrs. James' granddaughter, Kim, would come to visit her from California. My sister and I became good friends because we were either playing hopscotch outside in the yard or we would sit on her grandmother's porch as she showed us all of her Barbie dolls (that her grandmother purchased) and the chest full of clothes that she had for each of her dolls.

DETERMINATION

Kim and my sister Carolyn became very close during the summer I could remember one day when they suspiciously got their hands on some money and decided to walk to the convenience store that was couple of miles down Highway 80. I decided to sneak out of the house, and I followed them to the store. I waited outside until they came out.

Once they came out of the store, I noticed that they had two full paper brown bags of candy. I followed behind them. They walked very slowly down Highway 80 so that they could have enough time to eat as much of their candy before they made it back home. I tagged along behind begging for a piece of their candy as they shared their candy among themselves. Eventually, my sister gave me one piece of candy.

While I walked behind them, trying to remove the paper wrapping off the candy, my sister and Kim threw their bag of candy in the ditch and began to run down the side of the freeway very fast. I looked back and noticed the boys were following behind us. One of them was walking with a rope in his hand as a couple of them were riding on bikes.

"Run, Dee!" my sister screamed.

"What?" I asked with my mouth full of candy, not noticing the urgency.

"Run! If they catch you they going to tie you up to a tree and rape you!" she said. I looked back and noticed the boys begin to run behind us.

I start crying as I ran for my life, but I was barefooted. I didn't think to put on any shoes before I snuck out the house. The hard rocks on the side of the highway didn't bother my feet until I started running for my life.

My sister and Kim were putting a great distance between me and the boys who were just behind me. I used the balls of my feet to kick the rocks, but I still wasn't going any faster. Kim and my sister had turn the corner heading straight to our house, but I was still stuck behind crying and screaming at the same time. I was so afraid they would actually catch me, but as I looked back, they had stopped running. Once I got back to the house, I told my father about the incident, to which he thought they were just young boys playing around but to me they weren't.

If Kim wasn't visiting her grandmother doing the summer, we would normally play with our two friends that lived across the street from us. One of our friends, Brenda, didn't like to go home because she was having too much fun hanging out with us. Someone from her family would call out to her to come home because it was getting dark outside, but she would actually ignore them.

They stood outside begging her to come home but she wouldn't. She would stop and sit on our porch with her arms folded. "Brenda! Brenda, come—on home! It's getting late. It's time for you to come home, Brenda," they screamed across the street.

Sometimes, she would go home peacefully, but the majority of the time, she would fall on the ground and lay there kicking and screaming because she didn't want to go home. They had to actually walk across the street to our house and drag her from off of our porch or our front yard as we stood watching. They grabbed her arm and pulled her across the street, she'll fall to the ground again kicking and screaming until they finally picked her up and carried her inside of the house.

We had a lot of fun with Brenda, but we spent much of our time with our cousins in the country. Most of my father's family lived in Forkland, Alabama. We use to drive to Forkland a lot to visit them. I could remember the drive so well because I used to be so afraid of this large and narrow bridge—the Lake of Demopolis Bridge. The bridge had only two narrow lanes, and it stood so high. It made me so nervous every time my father drove across it!

Once we crossed the bridge, I would take a deep, relaxing breath, as we drove down the freeway. As we drove toward Forkland, there were a lot of trees and vacant land as far as I could see and there were homes that stood from the distance. A couple miles down the road, we passed a pool hall and a convenience store that stood next to one another. As my father drove up this little hill and around the curve, I could see from a distance the little white church we attended sometime.

Once we passed our church, we pass another large convenient store, as my father drove a couple of miles down the freeway. He would then make a right turn onto a two-lane road where there was a large black community. As he drove up the hill and around the sharp curve, I saw some of my grandparents' two hundred acres of land, where my father was born and raised on.

As we got closer to my cousin's house, my siblings and I sat up in our seats because we was so eager to get out the car so that we could have the best time of our lives playing with our cousins. My father drove up into their driveway, and our cousins rushed out of their house to greet us.

There were the six of us—my two sisters, my three cousins, and me. By them living on a farm, most of their chores were in the fields. At an early age, my cousins knew how to drive. I guess that by living in a rural area there wasn't much traffic in their small town. I used to sit on their front porch and watch my cousin, who was the same age as me, cutting their yard with the lawn tractor. Once they were finished with their chores, we would find fun things to do together. My oldest cousin, Ronnie, was our ringleader.

I admired my oldest cousin, Ronnie; he was very handsome. He was the one that stood out the most because of his great personality. People in general just loved him because he was so kind and had such a great sense of humor. I was excited to be in his presence. When Ronnie wasn't there when we came for visits, I never felt that we were having fun. It just didn't feel the same for me. Even though I loved my other cousins, he was my favorite.

Ronnie had such a beautiful singing voice. He sung mostly at church, but I never really got a chance to hear him sing solo at church because my family was always running late for church and by the time we got there the preacher was at the pulpit.

We didn't go to church every Sunday, but whenever we did, we all got dressed in our Sunday's best, and our father drove us to Forkland to attend Sunday services. As usual, we were always late. We had to stand in the corridor area until one of the ushers showed us to our seats, which by that time Ronnie had already sung.

After church, most of the time we would head straight or to our cousin's house. We would take off our church clothes and change into something so we could play outside. We sometimes gathered in their den to play our favorite records on their record player as we created a soul train line taking turns trying to see who could dance the best. Or we'd walk a mile down the road to the convenience store to purchase candy, ice cream, or Popsicles.

I always walked outside barefooted—even if the pavement was hot. We'll sometime walk down to our grandparents' house that was located in the back part of their large property a couple of miles down the road. As we walked toward their home, we always walked in the middle of the road. There was a small bridge we used to walk across, which I would normally walk across faster to avoid looking under the bridge.

Once we walked around the curve, I saw our grandparents' house. They had a very large house with a white picket fence that surrounded the front part of their house. Across the road was a lot of vacant land where their cattle grazed behind wired fences. There was a large barn a couple yards from their house, and on the side of the barn was a fence full of pigs.

As we got closer to their house, my grandparents would sometimes be sitting on their front porch. I would always take the time to notice the several berry trees that stood on the side of the house that I would sometime pull off to eat. We would walk up the steps, onto their large porch.

The entire porch was fully screened with two wooden swings on the opposite side of their porch. They had two doors, just a couple of inches apart, that we could use to enter their home, but I usually entered their house on the far right side of the porch. Sometimes our grandmother would be sitting in one of her swings as we walked onto the porch.

She was a very tall woman with a very smooth and fair complexion. Her voice was sort of deep and stern. She had raised six boys, including my father, and two girls. Most of my uncles and aunts lived in various states, but some lived close by. We definitely had a very large family.

As we walked onto the porch, we would give our grandmother a kiss on the jaw before entering their houses. I sometimes stayed outside with my two cousins as they took a stick from out of the yard to make a circle in the dirt to play marbles in the front yard of our grandparents' house, but most of the time, I followed my cousin (who was my age) to the kitchen.

Whenever we did enter their home, I would notice that the front room was very large but very dark. I could barely see anything but the fireplace that faced the front door that gave us a little light for navigating their home.

My grandparents had so many rooms in their large house, but as usual, we walked toward the kitchen, we passed another larger room where there was a large king size bed standing in the far left corner of the room. There was also a large fireplace that faced the bed that would be lit most of the time during the winter.

My grandmother watched us sometimes for our parents while they were at work or outings. Whenever we stayed overnight, I usually slept in the large room of the house where the fireplace was lit. During the cold mornings, I would wake up covered with at least two or more of my grandmother's homemade quilts. It would be so cold that I would just lie there, as my grandmother sat by the fireplaces to keep warm.

One morning, as I lay in bed, there was knocking at the front door. My grandmother sitting by the fireplace told whomever it was to come on in. A man walked in holding a dead possum. He greeted my grandmother, as he gave her the possum. I lay there watching my grandmother clean that possum with her bare hands over the hot burning fireplace. I thought for sure she was going to burn her hands as she pulled the hair off this dead animal's body, but it didn't bother her at all.

Later on that afternoon, I watched my grandfather as he sat humming a spiritual hymn as he sat in his hallway going up and down with both hands with a wooden plunger to churn buttermilk. I could put buttermilk in my cornbread, but I couldn't actually drink it because I didn't like the taste of homemade buttermilk. However, my younger cousin loved to drink it.

I use to follow him into the kitchen and watch him go into the refrigerator to get the container of buttermilk out as he reached into the kitchen cabinet for a glass. I watched him pour the chunky milk into a glass. I stood there frowning as he put the glass up to his lips and pull his head back so that he could get every drop down his throat.

I'd usually make myself a peanut butter sandwiches with some of my grandparents' homemade jam and sit at their dinning room table while I ate my sandwich. I would glance up at their painting of Tenth Commandments, trying to memorize each commandment so that I could use them at my parents' dinner table. "Thou Shall Not Steal; Thou Shall Not Have No Other God Before Me." The dinning room became one my favorite rooms in their house because I always got a chance to sit and learn at least one of the Commandments before I went home.

While our family lived in Demopolis, I attended their elementary school, which was a couple of miles from our house. Eventually, my father decided that my older sister and I should attend school with our cousins in Forkland. Every morning, my father dropped us off before he drove another ten minutes to Eutaw to teach his classes.

After school, my sister and I use to wait up front for our father to pick us up. If he was running late, we would play out front or be chased around the school by others kids as we waited. But if we weren't up front when our father arrived as he instructed there were consequences once we got home.

My father was strict and very consistent about the rules he set down for my sisters and I, which we would normally abide by. But as we gotten older, he became very protective when it came to his daughters. I can remember when my older sister went to her first prom at Forkland High School. My mother sewed my sister a beautiful gown for that special Saturday afternoon event. She pinned my sister hair up into a beautiful ball, and she drove her to Forkland and dropped her off at the school, while our father stayed at home cutting and attending his lawn.

I thought my sister looked so beautiful that day. Once my mother and I made it back home a couple of hours later, my father was finished cutting the lawn. He decided that we all would go to pick my sister back up. Once he arrived at the school, he parked his car in front of the school and got out. We waited in the car while our father went inside looking all dirty from working on the lawn. My sister came walking in front of our father with tears in her eyes.

My mother kept looking straight while not saying a word as my sister got in the back seat. We drove back across the bridge that Saturday afternoon with no one saying a word. I sat in the back seat looking at my sister's expression on her face. I knew she was so mad, disgusted, and totally embarrassed that our father actually walked into the prom looking the way he did as he pulled her out in front of all of her classmates when the prom had just started.

Whenever our father couldn't pick us up after school, my sister and I took the school bus to our grandparents' house, and we waited until our father got off work. While we waited for our father at our grandparent's house, I always knew when my father was outside because their dogs would be outside barking as he drove up toward our grandparents' house. I'll run outside on the front porch as I watched the dogs run around my father's car.

My father's got out of the car, and he walked to the back trunk of his car. He unlocks his trunk as he lift the trunk up and grabbed two buckets of food that was left over food from the high school cafeteria. As he poured the food into these large steel pan that were by the fences, the dogs rush over to the pans before my father could get all the food out of the bucket.

My mother's parents lived in Montgomery, Alabama. They would come to Demopolis to visit us sometimes. We were so excited to see them because they always bought us toys to play with whenever she came to visit. After staying for a couple of days, we always cried as they said their good-byes to us. As they back out of our driveway, we ran to the back porch to watch them drive down the Highway 80 as they headed toward home. Once we saw them on the freeway, they blew their horn as we stood on the back porch screaming as our parents tried to calm us down.

We would sometime take trips to Montgomery to visit them. It was a two-hour drive to Montgomery, but we didn't care because we were too excited that we were going to see our grandparents. As we drove toward Montgomery, there were a lot of small towns that we passed. I still to this day think that Alabama is a beautiful state with a lot of history behind it.

There was a lot of trees and old plantations that stood far in the distances as we sat in the backseat of our father's car. As we drove across Edmund Pettus Bridge in Selma, Alabama, our mother always reminded us of the struggle that took place here when she was very young. As we drove on, I knew when we had arrived in Montgomery city limits because we always passed by the city's airport at Dannelly Field on the right side of Highway 80.

DETERMINATION

We got very excited as our father drove into their community, which was kept up very well. It was an old predominately-black community; the yards and streets were clean where mostly everyone knew each other. Once my father made a left turn onto West Edgemont Street, he made another left onto McElvy Street. Soon, we could actually see our grandparent's front yard, where there was two large pine trees standing in the front yard as our father parked in front of their house.

We got out the car and walked onto the square cemented steps in their yard that lead us toward their front porch. My grandmother kept her yard cut and her scrubs trimmed neatly. As we got closer to the porch, I could see her beautiful red and white roses that were growing by the side of their house.

She greeted us at the front door as we entered their home. I always noticed a fresh smell as we walked through the door—like the famous perfume "White Castle." Everything was in its place. My grandmother had wonderful taste because most of her furniture had a contemporary style to it.

In the living room, she had a long tan sofa and two designer chairs that stood on the opposite side of the room. There was end tables on each side of the sofa with large lamps on each tables with little whatnots and ashtrays.

My grandmother enjoyed entertaining her friends when they came over for club meetings which she also enjoyed smoking a lot of "Camel Lights" cigarettes because I could also smell it once I walked into her house. There was a sofa table that stood by a very large window that outlook the roses that was growing on the side of her home. The curtains were in a tan color that brought a warm comfort as we entered their house.

By the window, there was a wooden shelf that stood in the corner that had various decorative accessories, but what really captured my sisters and my attention was the beautiful china doll that stood on the top of the shelf. We was so eager to touch that doll, but my grandmother had always put so much fear into us that we were too afraid to even get close to it.

My grandparents had a two bedroom home. The extra bedroom had a full size bed and an armoire that stood on the opposite side of their room. In their master bedroom, they had twin beds with the same silk comforter sets on their beds. Their television stood on the opposite side of the room against the wall in between their beds by the window as a cool breeze came through the open window. I would sit sometimes on the floor in their bedroom to watch *I Love Lucy* episodes.

As I sat there, the curtains were always pulled back so the breeze could come through the open window. I sat facing the window as the cool breeze hit my faces as I watched television. The breeze from the window was so strong that the tan silk curtains that covered my grandmother's large closet would move around where I was able to see all of her beautiful clothes she had.

I use to crawl on my knees and lie on my back as I put my head underneath the curtains as the wind blew the curtains in the air I'll peaked at all of her beautiful shoes and dresses she had stored in her closet. My grandmother worked as a maid for a very wealthy family in the north side of Montgomery. They thought a lot of her and gave her a lot of beautiful things that was hanging up in her closet and also in her home.

One summer while we were there visiting, our grandparents decided to have a barbecue in their backyard. We all sat down in folding chair talking and laughing while my father barbecued ribs. My grandfather's brother and our neighbors would come over to visit as we sat around in their backyard enjoying one another's company as my sisters and I played with our next-door neighbors who was around our ages. I remember my great-uncle coming over that day. He was my favorite uncle. As a child, I thought he was very tall; he would let me either jump on his back or shoulder just for the fun of it. He would carry me around and I felt like I could see forever.

Later on that day, our grandfather took us to the store, but it was actually a small brick house though it was set up as a store. There were shelves of candy and soda pops in freezer boxes. On the counter, there were jars of pig feet and pickles by the register, which I didn't like but my older sister did.

While our grandfather set talking with his friends, he let us chose whatever we wanted. We all got back in my grandfather's car, but as he drove up the hill headed back to his house, my little sister sat in the back seat with me while my older sister sat up front with my grandfather.

As we sat in the back seat, my little sister reached over the seats and put both of her hands over my grandfather's eyes while he was driving. My grandfather started to laugh as my sister made her stop. Once we made it back to our grandparent's house my sister told my father about what happened, but my parents didn't find the humor in it.

Whenever we came to Montgomery, our parents always took us to the country to visit our great grandparents that lived in a rural area of Pine Level, Alabama. My great-grandmother help raised my mother until my grandmother got herself situated in Montgomery, and my mother loved going down to see about her grandmother.

As we drove down Highway 231, I watched as my father turned onto this dusty and narrow road. There were a lot of trees, ditches, and old wooden bridges, but once we got to her house, there was a nice size pond that was a couple distance from their house. My great aunt lived pretty close by with her children, our cousins. She was younger than my mother, and they were very close because they basically grew up together.

While we were there, we mostly stayed outside and played with our cousins for a couple of hours as they sat on the front porch talking. I never forgot the little time that we did spend together that day because we were cousins, but we didn't see that much of each other because we lived so far away.

One summer, we stayed a week at our grandparents' house, and I could remember my grandmother taking us on picnics in the park. She would actually fix us lunches. As she placed our food in her lunch basket, she would ask one of us to carry a large thermal of punch to her car—an old 1960s' Chevy Oldsmobile. She drove us five miles to Oak Park. She sat at the picnic bench preparing our lunch, as we played on the playgrounds.

Some nights she would let me sit up late at night. While her and my grandfather lay in their beds, I would hear my grandfather—or sometimes my grandmother—snoring as I sat on the floor watching television. One night I sat up and watched Frank Sinatra and Kim Novak in the movie *Pal Joey*. That became my favorite movie, but as I got older, I begin to watch a lot of old movies that were produced back in the forties though the late sixties. I simply loved the history behind them.

My grandmother was a very pretty woman, who I thought had a lot of class. She was a very slim and tall and she kept her haircut very short and neatly taped in the back. Her haircut reminded me of the actress Jane Wyman in the *Magnificent Obsession*. I had a lot of respect for her because I knew exactly where I stood with her. She spoke her mind and she definitely didn't take any mess or nonsense from others either because she felt that they get respect when she received respect.

While we were there that summer, our grandparents left my older sister to watch us while she was at work. Our great aunt, who lived down the street walked down to our grandmother's house, asked if my sisters and I could come down to her house to peel some peas for her, which we did because we was taught to always respect our elders.

That entire afternoon we sat on her back porch with large bowls

DETERMINATION

in our laps as we peeled two bushel of peas. Once my grandmother got home, we asked her why our thumbs were purple after peeling peas. My grandmother was so mad because she was unaware that our aunt asked that of us. She got back in her car, and she drove down the street to our aunt's house, which was very apologetic afterward. My aunt has four children of her own, way older than us, who our grandmother thought could've pealed those peas not us.

My grandmother could be tough when she had to, and I think that's where I got a lot of my strength come from. When she said something, we listened—even my grandfather knew not to push my grandmother too far. She had a black shaggy dog that she named Honey. He was very playful at times, but he was very close to our grandmother.

Honey played with us for a while, but he usually laid next my grandmother's feet. It has been times that our grandmother warned us not to bother him if he didn't want to play because he would either growl at us. If we was too persistent, he would've us pinned up in a cornered showing all of his teeth, which scared the daylight out of me.

I had some wonderful memories with both of our grandparents, but there were other memories that I couldn't forget either as I was growing up. When I was getting older, I begin to be very afraid of my father. I loved him, but he made me nervous when I was around him.

As I got older, I realized that my father was happier and a delight to be around when he was drinking, but when he was sober, he was a very quite man. Sometimes, he'd walk in the house from a very hard day at work singing. I was excited to see the joy and the excitement on his face.

He would walk in with a brown paper bag in his hand as he went toward the kitchen to get a glass. In the bag, there was a bottle of liquor and a can of soda. Before we sat down to have dinner, our father would always sit in the living room in his black recliner chair, relaxing with a drink in one hand and a cigarette in the other.

That's when I noticed a lot of things I didn't like—especially the beatings that my mother went through. There were times that I couldn't go to sleep because I heard her cries late at night. I lay there listening to them through the whole ordeal, hoping for all of it to stop as my siblings slept peacefully.

I thought the world of my mother. She was beautiful. She was at least five foot four and small built. My mother had such a beautiful smile that was so warm. People enjoy simply being in her presences because she had such a great sense of humor. She loved to laugh and had gentleness about herself. She always put in that *special time* with us. I remember that when we were younger, she would actually sit with us and color in our coloring books. We would sometimes stop coloring and watch her color. We were so amazed how she stayed within the lines.

My mother loved my father so much, but sometimes the abuse could be too much for her. Various times she left our father, but she would eventually go back to him. As I got older, I sometimes wondered why she came back to him. I guess because of us.

One night my mother, my siblings, and I left with my aunt, and we didn't arrived back home until later on that night. When we arrived back, my aunt and uncle went inside our house and tried to calm our father down while my siblings and I sat in the car. I watched from in the back seat window of my aunt's car.

As I watched through the screen door, I sat there wondering if they would be able to calm my father down. I could tell my father was very anger with my mother. He sat in his chair not saying a word, facing my mother who sat across from him on the sofa.

He sat looking over at my mother. The only thing that was between the two of them was the coffee table, but I could tell by my mother posture she was so afraid to move. We sat in the car for a while, but as I sat there, I watched as my father immediately got up out of his chair, reached over the coffee table, and hit my mother.

I heard her screamed out loudly, and all of us rushed out of the car and ran into the house. There was blood everywhere leading into the kitchen, where my mother stood over the kitchen sink trying to stop the bleeding.

That night, they took my mother to the emergency room. Again, we sat in the car. The car windows were rolled down, but I could hear my mother's cries from the small window above where the car was parked.

After the incident happen, we stayed with my grandparents in Forkland for almost a week until my mother decided to go back home to my father. She didn't go to work for a week because her eye was black and blue, but whenever she had to run errands she worn sunglasses to hide her face.

Eventually, my father moved the family into a larger house. When we moved into our new home, I had my own room, located on the other side of the house by the kitchen area. I was so afraid to go to sleep at night because it was so dark, and I was all alone in that back room. I would just lie in bed and look out the bedroom window at the lights that coming from across the street that came from the top of the hill.

As I lay there, I wondered what was up on that hill—until one day my sister and I decided to climb the hill. We saw a baseball field with lights that lit the entire baseball field and the surrounding area. There were people who stood out in the field while people were sitting on the bleachers watching and cheering for their team.

The following year our family moved again; this time, we lived a couple blocks from a Baptist church. My siblings and I would walk to church to attend Bible study and Sunday services. There was a funeral home not that far from our house, which I could actually see it from out of my bedroom window.

At the time, I was afraid of funeral homes especially after I jumped in the back seat of my aunt's car after Sunday services in Forkland. Not asking where we were headed because all I wanted to do was to hang out with my cousin. My aunt drove down the narrow dirt road to a small house that stood near the road.

We all got out of her car and walked up the steps, and as they open the door, I noticed caskets in the front room. It was too late; I couldn't turn around because my cousin was behind me. I walked in, and there were at least six caskets in the room—an entire family who had died in a car accident.

The family was headed home from church as they were hit in a head-on collision because two guys were drag racing on a two-lane road. I stood there unable to move after I saw an infant lying in a very small casket with his family. Once we left, I was so scared and sadden by the loss of the family. That day changed me! I learned how to appreciate my life more.

Things were getting worse at home, especially between my parents, but as I was getting older, I understood what was going on. Unfortunately, I wasn't able to forget the beatings and still had trouble sleeping at night because I could still hear my mother's cries as they came from across the hallway.

I begin to notice that whenever my siblings went to visit my grandparents in Montgomery, I was left behind with my parents. I thought at first that my grandmother didn't want me there, but I began to realize that I was there with my mother for a reason. I used to sit in my room and wonder if I did something wrong, asking why my siblings were in Montgomery and why was I stuck in Demopolis with my parents.

One evening as I played in my room, my mother came in to tell me that one of our childhood friends, Brenda's brother who lived in our old community, had died in a car accident. He was one of the siblings who use to drag Brenda off our porch or insisting she needed to come home.

My mother told me that his body was around the street at the funeral home. She asked me if I wanted to walk over to view his body. I immediately told her "no" because I wanted to remember him how he was when I was little. Plus, I was scared and too shocked over his death. I didn't want to remember him lying up in a casket.

That evening my father came home. Both of my parents were in their bedroom when I heard my father screaming and hitting my mother for not flushing the toilet. I sat on the edge of my bed as I listen to her cries as he hit her. But something came over me that night. I walked out of my room into the hallway and stood there until I got the courage to slowly walk toward their bedroom.

I stood at their doorway, not sure if I should say anything because I was afraid of him but I just didn't want him to hit her anymore. I couldn't stand to hear my mother cry either. I looked over at my mother as she laid across the bed curled up in a knot while my father stood over her.

"Don't hit her no more!" I screamed. He turned toward me with shock on his face. I didn't know what was about to happen to me and I didn't care.

He walked up to me. "You don't understand, Dee," he said. When you get older, you'll understand.

I started crying while I looked up at my father. "Please don't hit her anymore, Daddy, please," I said.

That night the house was silent. I went back to my room and sat in the dark on the edge of my bed. I stared out the window not knowing what was going to happen next. All I knew that it was peaceful that night, and I didn't hear my mother's crying.

As I sat there in the dark, I looked across the street at the funeral home thinking about my friend who I grew up with and how my father beat me so badly once that he left a sore on my side as I tried to get away.

One day, my parents left me to babysit my sister. We were two years apart, but we were older enough to stay at home. After my little sister had poured cooking grease on the floor, I tried to mop it up, which only made it worst. But once my parent's arrived home that night my father noticed how slippery and sticky the kitchen floor was.

I tried to explain to my father what had happen, but I was so young at that time and didn't realize that I should've used soap and water to clean up the grease rather than smudging the grease around with the mop. My father was very upset with me. He began to pull his belt from his pants, as I began to back up begging him not to spank me.

As he got closer to me, I ran and he chased me around the house in a circle, while hitting me with his belt. I begged him to stop, as I tried to get away from him. I kept screaming that I didn't do it, but he wouldn't stop until I said I made the mess on the kitchen floor.

My mother left him after that beating, and she took us to live with our grandparents in Montgomery. My mother pulled my shirt up to show my grandmother the scar he left on my side from chasing me throughout the house.

My mother moved us out of our grandparents' house into the projects, which was an adjustment for us all. Things were very hard for our mother because she was taking on a big responsible by taking care of four children with only one income.

For the first time she had to use food stamps just to put food on our table. Things were really hard for our mother even though she was able to keep her same job—they transferred her to their plant in Montgomery.

My older sister was older enough where she could watch us while my mother went to work at the plant. My mother had economized by buying fabric and patterns from the store to sew our clothes for school or for special events at church. I used to watch her as she laid fabric on the floor and pinned the patterns to the fabric before she neatly cut them out before sewing them together.

She brought a sofa and love seat from a friend for our living room. She went out and bought two large rolls of dark floral printed of fabric so that she could re-upholster the furniture. This was my mother's personal and special project and she worked very hard on it. I watched as she and my sisters ripped the old fabric from the bases of the sofa and love seat and sewed and staple the new fabric onto the sofa and love seat.

Within a year, my mother decided to go back to my father. We moved back into the same house and my mother used her furniture, including the sofa and love seat that she personally re-upholstered, to decorate the living room.

Soon things began to get rocky in their relationship again. One night my mother was too afraid to go home because she knew my father was at home waiting for her. We all walked with our mother to her best friend's house because she was afraid to face our father, but it was getting late so we all finally decided to walk home.

Once we got closer to the house, we noticed that our father's car was in the driveway. My mother slowly walked up the steps onto the porch as we followed behind her. The door was open and our father was sitting in the living room waiting for her in his black recliner.

As she slowly opened the screen door and entered the living room, she noticed that my father had cut the skirts of her sofa (that she worked hard to re-upholster) with a razor. My mother stood at the door, crying and breathing really hard.

She picked the broom up that was standing in the corner and tapped him on the shoulder. As she dropped the broom on the floor, she ran out the front door. We followed behind our mother like little chicks following their mother hen. Our little dog followed behind us as we followed our mother down the street.

    She begin to walked back to her friend's house that we had just left, but as we were walking across the street, our little dog got hit by a car that night. We stood at the curve crying over his death, but our mother continued on her mission. Once my mother arrived at her friend's house, she called the police, and they arrested my father that night. While he was sitting in jail, my mother went back to the house, packed all our things, and she drove his car back to Montgomery that night. She never looked back again.

PUTTING MY LIFE IN PERSPECTIVE

After my mother went back home, James and I decided to move into separate bedrooms because we were getting into a lot of silly arguments. Since Lauren was staying in Florida until I got better, I decided to move into my daughter's bedroom. I move all of my personal belongings including my clothes into her closet.

I drove myself to the clinic in Plano every other day for platelet, fluids, and blood transfusion so that I could build up my immune system for my next chemotherapy treatment. I would sit behind a curtain with a little television as I watched other cancer patients get their own treatment.

While I was at the clinic, one of the nurses took me in one of the bathrooms so she could show me how to clean and flush my Hickman line. She insisted that I took my shirt off so that she could explained and show how to used syringe to flushed and cleaned the two tubes. That scared the daylights out me, but I was also embarrassed because I didn't want her to see my scar on my chest or any part of my body.

In due time, my head was bald. I wore a wig. But it just didn't feel comfortable, so every time I had to go to the clinic, I wrapped a scarf around my head and a baseball cap to hide my head and face. When I got home, I walked around bald; my head was always cold.

I received a letter from my mother once she made it back home. I open it and I read it:

Hi,

Your momma has been praying for you. If you need me, I'll be there for you. I will pay my way. I remembered when you were six or seven years old. When your father started fights with me, you would always there telling him, "Don't you hit my momma."

You have always been close to me; he felt like you loved me more than him because the others never open their mouths. You will always be my baby. I don't know if you thought my heart wasn't big enough to love all of you. You can't do anything to stop me from loving you. I won't say anything ugly to you. You know it, but you push me too far sometimes. The minute I say it, God makes me humble.

Love Momma.

I felt bad the way we left. I decided to call her and asked her to forgive me. She told me she loved me, and if I needed her to come back down to let her know. She came straight out and told me that she didn't care for James. It was something sneaky about him, whom I agreed with her, but it was too late. I had to deal with him until my lease came up.

On October 9, 1997, while I was at home, I received a large envelope in the mail from the National Bone Marrow Registry. There was a brochure and letter informing me that I was put on the National Registry lists. *How? I thought the doctor wasn't going to put me on the registry.* But somebody did.

I admitted myself back into the hospital so that I could start on my second set of chemotherapy for that week. When the nurse pulled the chemical from the container, the fluid was red fluid. She told me some of the side effects as she gave me a piece of paper that explained more into details about the procedure.

I read some of the side effects of the chemical that was called Idarubxcin. It stated that it caused urine to turn reddish in color, which may stain clothes. If the medication accidentally seeps out of the vein, it might damage some tissues and cause scarring.

While I went through a week of chemotherapy, I gargled twice a day so that I wouldn't get sores in my mouth during each treatment. I never had any flare ups or any sores, which I thought was a blessing.

After my treatment, they had to do another biopsy to see if the treatment put me in remission, but I wasn't. I stayed in the hospital for another week until my white blood cell was up so that my immune system was able fight off infections.

While I was still in the hospital, I had more blood transfusion and platelets. Not once did James visit me. I got to the point I didn't care anymore, I knew that I had to go through this fight alone.

James would call periodically, but we didn't have that much to say to one another. I decided to call him just to see if everything was okay at home. "My mother's here," he said.

"She's where?" I asked.

"She's here in Dallas. She came on the bus unannounced."

"Oh, really?"

"Yea," he said.

He took a sigh of relief. "DD, when I got there she was at the bus station, she had all these boxes that was stack to the top of ceiling."

"What were they?" I asked.

"It was a lot of her personal items that she brought down with her. She's still insisted on us moving in my own apartment so that we can be together as a family."

"Where is she?"

"She's in their laying down right now."

"Laying down where?" I asked.

"In my bedroom," he said.

"In our apartment?"

"Yes."

"I'm sorry James, but I don't want her there because all the things that you told me about your mother. Why all of sudden did she come down when I got sick? Plus, she doesn't like me," I said.

"I know, DD," he said.

"James to be honest with you, I think that you need to get your own apartment for yourself and your mother because she doesn't have anybody or anywhere else to go. That's your mom," I said.

He didn't say anything for a while, but all of sudden, he told me that they were trying to sell his mother's house. I was still clueless as to why would they sell her house if she didn't have anywhere to live or go?

After I got off the phone, I felt bad because I was being selfish toward his mother, but I didn't trust James anymore than I trusted his mother. Mostly everything in the apartment was mine, and I worked hard for what I had. I didn't want to lose it by people I didn't know.

The only true friend I could talk to was Horace. He called me everyday whether I was in the hospital or at home. I met him when we worked at the law firm. We became quick friends. He was so funny, and he had such a great sense of humor. He made me laugh and I could always be myself with him.

Even when times were very hard for both of us, we were there for each other. He was like a brother to me. He was my best friend. When he first found out I had Leukemia, he immediately brought it upon himself to locate a clinic so that he could get his blood tested to see if he had the same blood protein as mines.

After he left the clinic, he called me and told me that he set up a date and time to go in to be tested during the week. I thought it was so nice of Horace to take the time and effort to get himself tested for me because he didn't have to. After that, I began to question James's affection for me. Several months had passed, and he hadn't taken the initiative to go into a clinic to get tested. *Why?* I asked myself. *I thought that he loved me. Was he afraid of the unknown or does he even love me like he said?*

Some of my coworkers, who were my close friends and Caucasian that called and asking where they could go to get tested. I had to turn around and tell them they couldn't because our protein in our blood was different proteins, and I need a donor from my own race.

During my doctor's visit, he informed me they asked that my sibling to go in to one of the clinics in Montgomery to get tested, but they haven't gone in yet. He couldn't understand why, and I couldn't either. If it was one of them, I would've gone in by then, but obviously, they had their own personal reasons why it was taking them so long to get tested. *Was it something that I said or done? Or did it have something to do with me leaving and moving to Texas? Or maybe they were unclear how serious this disease was.* I didn't have the answers.

While I was in the hospital, I thought it was sort of strange that when I talked to my African American friends about me needing a bone marrow transplant to prolong my life they told me that they would pray for me—with the exception of Horace. I couldn't understand why there so much fear especially with my family, I thought we were close we had all these wonderful memories together. I was stunned.

My mother did a great job keeping us together as a family once she moved us to Montgomery. My mother eventually divorced our father. We lived with our grandparents in Mobile Height for a little while until my mother rented a three-bedroom house across Freeway 65, not far from our grandparents' home. One morning my mother came into our bedroom and told us that our grandmother had passed away. I didn't think that much of it until we were sitting in a limousine with our father that was parked in front of the church.

While my sisters and I looked through the window, I watched, with my family as my grandmother's friends and family gathered in front of the church to show their respect and love as they took her casket inside. It all came to us that we weren't going to see her again. We started to cry as we looked on while my little brother was constantly asking our father why we were crying. My brother was too young that he really didn't understand all of the wonderful memories we had shared with our grandmother.

During the services, the intermediate family had to go up and view her body for the last time, but when the time came and my mother walked up toward her casket, she fainted. We sat there and crying, as my father picked my mother up and carried her outside. We trailed behind the hearse to the gravesite in the country where they laid my grandmother to rest and said our final good-byes to her.

My grandfather asked my mother to move us into his home after he finished remodeling his house to add on additionally rooms for us. During the reconstruction, my grandfather had a major stroke that left him paralyze on his left side. My mother decided to move in immediately into our grandfather's house so that she could take care of him once he was out of the hospital. He never had a chance to really finish remodeling his home; there was a lot of work that needed to be done.

Once we moved into our grandfather house and got him situated in one of the remodeled rooms, we unfortunately found out that there were a lot of problems with the house. We began to notice that whenever it rained the house flooded. We would sometimes wake up the next day where the carpet was soaked through.

There has been a time when we would wake up with an inch of

water in the house, which eventually destroyed the new carpet my grandfather put down during reconstruction. We decided we had to pull the carpet up because it began to smell awful. We were lucky because there was tile underneath the carpet.

The locks on some of the bedroom doors were installed outside of the room rather than inside, and the windows were installed upside down. But my mother mainly was concern with the flooding. She had to call out various contractors to give her an estimate and to also figure out why our house would flood after a massive storm.

Eventually, one contractor found out what was the problem; he explained to our mother that we lived on a street that has a hill and where our house stood, which was in the middle, the rain in the end would settled and ended at our home house due to bad construction work.

My mother paid the contractor to fix the problem, but by this time, she was up to her neck in debts. She eventually took out a loan to cover for various repairs that needed to repair to our home, but she also had to put the house up as collateral to get this loan, which made it even more difficult for her to pay other bills.

One day, as I walked into the house, I noticed my mother sitting on the couch crying as this man sat next to her holding her hand comforting her.

"Momma, are you okay?" I asked. She nodded her head saying yes, as I went back to my room wondering what happen, but I eventually found out later that the bank had sold our house to the gentleman that sat next to her that day.

Regardless of the outcome, we were still very excited that we moved into my grandparents' house because there were a lot of fun memories that we shared there. The community was a very close net. Everyone practically knew one another, and we had a majority of older neighbors who had been in the community for years, which was a good thing because it brought more moral values to the community. The people were very friendly too.

Sometimes I would sit on the edge of the curve in the front of our house and watch some of the boys in our community play catch football in the middle of street until the streetlight came on because we all knew we had to be inside the house by that time.

When my mother purchased her first car (a light blue Buick Regal), she was so excited that she gathered us all into her new car and drove us to the country to see our great-grandmother to spend some time with our cousins too. Almost every weekend she would take us down to see them.

During the summer time, my mother loved driving us to the country. My siblings and I often fought over who was going to sit in the front or by the window. I would normally sit in the back seat with the windows down as our mother drove us down the Highway 230.

As the breeze hit my face, I'll look out the window at the long and lonely road as we drove across small bridges with small lakes underneath as we headed down the freeway toward Pine Level. I always noticed large green trees, standing a short distance away from the highway.

As the wind hit my face, I begin to wonder how lonely it might be for some people who decided to live so far away from the city. *What if they had an emergency?* I thought, and I wondered how long it would take an ambulance to come in case of an emergency.

We passed this farm where large trees that hidden this very large field of crops. This particular farm stood not that far from the freeway. I could clearly remembered that field because my cousin had put in my head that we could make a lot of money picking peas on that particular farm that my mother just passed by.

I looked over at the farm, I thought about the phone call I received from my cousin asking if I wanted to make some extra cash over the summer. I was excited. I was going to work for the first time, and I would actually have my own money. I bragged to my siblings that

I was going to make a lot of money picking peas at a farm near my great-grandmother's house because hard work didn't bother me. I asked my mother to drop me off one weekend so that I could spend a week with my cousin, which she did.

That Monday morning, we woke up around dawn the sun was barely out. We got dressed and quickly ate breakfast before someone came to picked us up for work. I heard someone blowing a horn in front of my cousin's house. We both ran to the front door where we noticed it was a pickup truck.

My cousin closed the front door. We ran toward the pickup as the man waited for us to get in the back of the truck where there was others who he had picked up who were already sitting or standing in back of his truck. "Come on," my cousin said. We both got in the back, and I sat next to my cousin, as the farmer drove further down the dirt road to pick up more people to pick his crops.

Once he picked up several other people, he drove back onto Highway 230. I held on for dear life, as I sat back there thinking, *How did I get myself into this? What was I thinking about?* I asked myself. Once he drove through wired fence and up toward his farm, I noticed he had a lot of land, filled with peas that need to be picked.

When he stopped and parked the truck, we all jumped out the back of his truck. I was excited once again. My cousin told me to follow her, which I did.

"Get one of those baskets," she said.

"Okay." I said. I picked up a very long and large basket that was very light that I could actually carry it with one hand. I followed my cousin toward the field so that she could show me exactly what I needed to do, but as we walked down an isle, I noticed rows and rows of peas that we had to pick.

"Come on Dee," she said.

"Oh okay," I said. I kept thinking *that this doesn't look too easy.*

"Now what do we suppose to do again?" I asked my cousin.

"We have to pick these peas and fill up both of our basket to the top and then he'll pay us at the end of the day."

"Oh—okay."

I took my basket and kneeled down as I begin to pick the peas, but I noticed the other workers were pretty fast. They were going down the rows pretty fast as they picked peas. The sun was beaming down in my face as the day went on. It became so hot that we took breaks under the only shade we had, which was under a couple small trees that stood against the wired fences next to the farmer's field.

We were out there for hours working so hard, trying to fill up those two large baskets before the end of the day. The bugs were biting my legs, and I had to constantly fight them off, especially the ants. They were having a field day because I had on shorts and Ked tennis shoes.

Whenever we took a break from being in the hot sun, we sat under that tree, trying figure out how long we had to do this because we were exhausted. Soon, we realized we were almost finished filling up the two baskets with peas.

I thought for sure he would probably pay us pretty good since we were out there for hours in the hot sun picking peas for him. Maybe the other workers who had more experience would definitely get paid more but only because it didn't take them as long as it took us to fill our baskets up. All I knew at the end of the day was I was so tired and I wasn't going to do this again, ever!

Once we filled up our baskets to the top, we got in a line with the others workers and waited until it was our turn for the farmer to put our baskets on the scales. When we got up there, he put one basket at a time on the scale. He sat both of the baskets to the side. He reached down into his cash box and began to count his money. He put seven dollars in my cousin's hands. "Thank you." she said.

I looked at him, and I looked at her like, *where's the rest?* I didn't say anything because I was too tired and hot and sticky from working hard in the sun. I just wanted to get back to my aunt's house so that I could take a bath and set under a fan.

I jumped back on the truck thinking to myself, *You fool!* I looked at my cousin.

Is this it? I asked.

"Yes," she said. We'll divide the money when we get home.

"Huh? Like what money?" I said to myself. I enjoyed hanging with my cousin but Uh-uh. I stood and bend all day in that hot sun picking peas, and at the end of the day, I only got paid $3.50?! It was no way I was going to do this again.

When he dropped us off in front of my aunt's house, I went in, took a bath, and lay across the bed because I was sick and disgusted by the little money we made. I mean I was actually sick.

I called my mother at work to see if she could come down to pick me up once she got off work, which she did. Once she arrived, I headed straight into my mother's car. When my mother arrived at my aunt's house, she got out of her car to talk with my aunt, who was sitting on her back porch. I pulled the passenger seat back as far as I could as I lay there like a sick dog while my mother sat talking to my aunt for hours. I didn't care what they said; I just wanted to go home.

For many years, my siblings teased me about that particular day. They would sometimes reminded me by laughing and saying, "Dee, you remember when you went to the country thinking you was going to make a lot of money picking peas and you came back with $3.50?" At first, I was ashamed, but as I got older, I began to appreciated those time that I spent with my cousin on that hot day because I learned that everything that sounds good doesn't mean that it's good and that sometime you have to work a little harder.

As my mother got closer to our great-grandmother's house, I could see the filling station on the right sided of the highway that we always passed before we made a right turn heading toward our great-grandmother's house. There would be people standing in front of the store talking or putting gas in their cars. I would sometimes walk back up to the store with our cousins to purchase candy or just to hang out for a little while as we watched people play pool.

Once she made a right turn onto the dirt road, there was a house that stood behind the store. As we proceed down the road, there was a small abandon house that stood on the opposite side of the road. She then made a left turn onto a very small and narrow dirt road.

As we made a left turned onto another road, I would look through the back window of my mother's car to see if any of my cousins were playing on their front porch or in the yard. On the left side of the road, there a small shotgun house, and across the road was an old farm, where a cotton gin stood in the middle of field. The road was very bumpy road as we headed toward our great-grandmother's house. Whenever my mother's tires would hit a bump or a hole in the road, our bodies would jump up and down.

As we got closer to her house, I could see my great-grandmother looking through her side window as we drove up. She came out of her house and walked to the edge of her porch to greet us. During summer days, I noticed that she always wore very soft cotton printed dress that kept her cool doing the hot days.

Once my mother parked the car and we all got out, I took my shoes off so that I could feel the soft and soothing tan color sand that was in the front of her yard. I would actually stand outside sometimes and just to walk around in the sand barefooted, as the sand ran through my toes.

As my great-grandmother stood waiting on her front porch, we would walk up the steps and give her a kiss on the jaw before we walked onto the porch. My great-grandmother was a very tall, slim, and a beautiful black woman. She didn't look her age because her skin was so beautiful and very smooth

As we walked into her house, I felt a fresh cool breeze as I entered the front door. Her television stood against the wall by the front door and the window as I walked in. She had two beds that stood on opposite sides of the room.

Her fireplace was on the right side of the room where there were two wooden chairs that stood next to the fireplaces. My great-grandmother's chair was always next to the window so that she could see who was passing through or as we came toward her house.

I would pass through the front room headed straight toward the kitchen, where there stood, in the far right side corner, an old wood burning stove. There always seemed to be food cooking on top of the stove and cornbread sitting in the top shelf of the stove.

Once I passed through the kitchen, I walked outside to the back porch. There was a small chicken house that stood far away in her backyard. As I walked down the steps, where there was a path that I would sometimes follow my cousins down to fetch water from the well. Whenever we walked down the path into the woods, I would always stand farther away from the well as they filled buckets with water. I was too afraid to get near the well because they told me if anyone ever fell in there they would've drown because it that deep.

I enjoyed spending time in the country with our cousins; we had so much fun together. Whenever there was a special event at our great grandmother's church, my mother would sometime get us all dress early on Sunday morning. She then drove to Pine Level to attend her church with her grandmother. The church was an old white wooden house with a temple on top of the roof. It stood a couple of miles from the highway and was hidden off by large trees that our mother would always park under for shade during the hot summers.

During some of the church services, we would sit in our Sunday best as we tried to keep cool with little cardboard fans while the preacher preached the word of the day. There was one air conditioner but most of the breeze came through the open windows. After church members prepared a fest for a particular special event, they would serve the food outside under the shade where it was cool.

After church, we went back to our great-grandmother's house and played outside with our cousins in the sand in her front yard while the adults sat on the porch talking until it was dark outside. Eventually my mother and my great grandmother would go inside of the house as it got darker outside. I would sometime sit and listen to them talk in the dark next to the fireplace as they discussed who died or got shot or stabbed and who put hoodoo on someone, which scared the daylight out of me.

My cousins would sometime walk down to our great-grandmother's house late at night. They weren't afraid of the dark because they were use to it but not for me, I was too afraid. It reminded me of my favorite movie, *The Shepherd of the Hills,* where Betty Field had to walk in the woods late at night to get to Harry Carey's house.

I sat there listening to them talking, and I thought, *No way am I going to sleep after listening to all of these stories!* I was definitely not going to sleep not until we were back in Montgomery and my mother was in our driveway. I honestly felt that my mother knew I was afraid and that's why she always had me sitting up front on the passenger side whiles my sisters and brother were in the back seat asleep.

I barely blinked my eyes while she drove back up toward the highway. I looked around at everything wondering who was going to pop out of the trees. Once we drove up toward the front entry where there was light, my mother would normally make a right turn headed home, but if it wasn't too late she made a left turn to stop by our great aunt's house where we enjoyed many wonderful memories together.

When we're at home, we spent a lot of our time with our friends in the community, but our mother wanted to know exactly where we were at all times; she didn't play when she say that we had to be home before the street lights came on. If we weren't there, she would actually come looking for us. Or she would wait until we walked into the front door, and there were consequences to pay.

One day she told us in advance to be at home early one evening because she had a club meeting to go to, and she didn't want to worry about us while she was away. We were expected to be at home before she left for her club meeting, but my little sister thought otherwise.

My sister was down the street playing with one of our friends at the time, as my mother was still getting dress. She waited for a while on the porch with me to see if maybe my sister would eventually come home on her own, but that never happened. She went back into the house as I stood on the front porch with my brother. Soon, our mother walked out of the house, and she told us *not* to go anywhere while she was gone.

As she was walking toward her car, I noticed she had her purse in one hands and a belt in the other. She backed her car out of the driveway, and she drove a couple houses down the street to where my sister was playing inside our friend's house.

She parked her car in the front of their house. She got out the car as she wrapped her belt twice around her hands and walked toward their front door. She knocked on the glass door. Once the front door opened, my sister greeted my mother at the door, as she slowly walked out their house. When she saw that my mother had a belt in her hands, she slowly backed up. My mother grabbed her by the arm and turned her around and gave her couple of licks on the behind, as she pointed toward our house.

My sister walked toward our house crying, but mostly it was just her feelings that were hurt and embarrassed. I watched my mother get back in her car and drove down the street. As my sister walked on the porch, I stood there laughing. But the apple didn't fall too far from the tree. My mother had greeted my older sister or me at the door for coming through the window because we came home after our curfew.

As we got older, there were more punishments than spankings. My mother had rules, and we were going too abided by them. When she called out for us, we always said, "Yes, ma'am!" or "No, ma'am!" It was never "What?" I did that once, and I never did it again. She raised us to respect others and especially our elders.

She taught us how to be compassionate toward others and treat them, as we wanted to be treated. She told me once if I told a lie once I would have to tell another lie to cover up the first lie so why not tell the truth so that it could save a lot of drama.

My mother and brother had such a wonderful relationship with one another that as I look back there were some wonderful and funny memories. I could remember during the spring when our mother love to do a lot of spring cleaning. She had my little sister and I inside the house cleaning up while she and my brother and one his friend was outside racking leaves into various piles in the backyard before she burned them.

While my sister and I were in the house cleaning, all of sudden, we heard a loud boom! My sister and I ran to the front door, trying to figure out where the sound came from, but we didn't see anything until we saw our brother running very fast from the side of the house and into the street headed up McElvy, as his friend ran behind him.

As we watched them run up the street. "Get him Buster! Catch him!" My mother screamed as she ran toward the house.

"I need my car keys!" she screamed. Get my car keys! We ran into the house and we got her keys.

"Give me the keys," she said.

"What happen, mamma?" I asked.

"Your brother put a spray can in a pile of burning leaves and he almost blew my head off."

She immediately got into her car and backed out of the drive

DETERMINATION

way headed up the street trying to catch up with my brother. I don't remember if she spanked him, but my mother had a great sense of humor, and she could be so funny whenever she got angry with him or with anyone. It got to the point that I couldn't do anything but laugh because my mother had a way of expressing herself whenever she called him or us out our names.

One evening, my little brother and I went to the grocery store with our mother to buy self-rising flour for a cake she was trying to bake. My mother drove my oldest sister's white Volkswagen Bug to the store, as I sat in the back seat with my feet up on the side of the floor because there was a large hole in the floor of my sister's car. I could actually see the pavement from the street as my mother drove us to the grocery store.

Once we arrived at the store, my mother parked the car, as she looked at both of us. "So—which one of you is going inside the store for me?" she asked.

"Me!" my brother said.

"Okay, Scotty," she said. I need self-rising flour to bake my cake.

"Okay, Momma."

My mother reached into her purse and she gave my brother the money, but as she put the money in his hand, she looked over at him as he opened the car door.

"Okay, Scotty," she said. I need self-rising flour.

"Okay...Momma," he said.

As my mother and I sat waiting patiently for my brother to come out of the grocery store, she noticed him walking toward the car with a shopping bag in his hand. My mother tried to start the car but it wouldn't start. She pressed down on the gas a little, as she played around with the clutch but the car still wouldn't start.

As my brother opened the door and sat down on the passenger side, my mother grabbed the bag out of his hand and looked into the bag and she stared at my brother.

"I told you self-rising flour!" she said. "You went straight in that store and got the regular flour." She gave the bag back to him as he pulled out a Crunch N' Munch candy bar out of the bag that he bought with the extra changes that was left over.

I sat in the back seat shaking my head and smiling because I knew my mom was going to give him a mouth full once she got the car started. She was still trying to get the car started, but it wouldn't. She pressed down on the gas pedal and turning the ignition, but it still wouldn't start.

We sat there quietly in the parking lot wondering if the car would ever start. I could tell she was getting a little frustrated but as we all sat quietly in the car while my brother sat crunching on his candy bar. I look over at my mother who was already frustrated with my sister's car as she constantly kept messing around with the clutch.

She waited for a second. It became totally quiet in the car except for the sound of my brother crunching and smacking on his candy, which I became very tickled that I start laughing. I knew eventually my mom was going to let him have it.

She looked over at him. "Scotty, I told you to go inside the store and get me the self-rising flour, but you come back with what I told you *not* to get and now you sit over there smacking like a damn horse!" she said. I start to laugh even harder.

My mother turned around and looked back at me. "Shut up Dee!" she said.

"Scotty, one day you're going to take some young lady out to dinner and she going to get up and leave you right there once she hear how you chew your food," she said. It's a damn shame you smack like that!

By this time I was down in the back seat laughing so hard that I had totally forgot about the car not starting. We sat there for a while until eventually she got the car to start, but I had some wonderful

Determination

and funny times with my family because my mother could be the funniest person even when she wasn't trying to be.

We joke and made fun of each other, which we would laugh at some of the dumb things we've done in the past, which we had a specific way of saying or expressing ourselves rather than being upset, which we learned from her. People in our neighborhood would drop by our house just to get a good laugh after getting off work and before they went home for that day.

Growing up, I really admired my oldest sister. She had so much patience and calmness about herself. It took a lot to get her upset. She had invited me to go with her to this nightclub that was downtown. She gave me her keys that night, and she asked me if I would go to her car and to get something for her, which I did, but when I put her key in the door to unlock her Volkswagen, I accidentally broke the key in the lock.

I stood outside in the cold for a while because I was so afraid to go back into club to tell her what had happen. I thought for sure she was going to kill me. Finally, I got up the nerve to go back in to tell her what had happen because she was going find out anyway.

As I walked back in the club, I told her what had happen, and she was very calm about the hold incident. She actually had an extra key in her purse, which she used to open the passenger door to get in which I was so relieved.

I was in the sixth grade when I first attended Carver High School that was located in our community; I use to walk to school every morning. Once I was in the twelfth grade, it was really time for me to get serious about my future and what I wanted to do with my life after high school. I begin to understand that each classes that I chosen was very essential that I passed if I wanted to graduated on time. I learned that I did well when I took hard classes because they were a challenge to me.

There was one class that I dread taking—Driving Education. I was so afraid to drive, but I knew I had to take the class if I wanted to graduate. I remember sitting in this class and having to sit in a booth with a picture screen that stood in front of us with a steer wheel and a gas pedals and brakes underneath our feet.

I was awful in that class! The teacher began to show the class various films on the projector on how it was important to pay attention while driving. It got to the point that it begin to bother me a lot because the films were so explicit in details. I sat in my desk with my head down or my hands over my eyes.

The films were showing the aftermath of the accident, too; that really freaked me out. It was so dramatic that I was screeching in my desk and making awful noises as the other students started laughing. My teacher had enough. He walked over to my desk and picked up the desk while I was still sitting and turned my desk toward the wall, while the students laughed and went back watching the rest of the film.

Eventually, my teacher had to take two students at a time out into the community to teach us some of the basics of driving a car and to see what we had learned in his classes. I was up first, while the other student sat in the back seat. When I got in the driver's seat, I was so nervous, but I did exactly what he told me to do. I put my seat belt on first and checked my front and side rear view mirrors before I started the car.

As I put my foot on the brakes, I started the car and put the car in drive. I drove through the school parking lot where I stopped at the stop sign. My teacher told me to make a right turn onto Oak Street. I put my right signal on before I made a right turn. I slowly made a right turn off the school campus. As I proceed into my community, I was driving at least twenty-five miles per hour before he told me to make a right turn onto Potomac Street.

Once I turned on Potomac Street, I went up the hill, where I came to a complete stop at the railroad track. I looked both ways as we went across the railroad track. Once I stopped at the stop sign on Boone Street, he asked me to make a left turn. As I turned onto

DETERMINATION

Boone Street, I drove down the hill, and I noticed we were getting closer to the end of the street. My teacher asked me to come to a complete stop. Once I got to the stop sign, I could only make either a right or left turn on West Edgemont Avenue because there were homes facing us.

But once I got to the stop sign, I had to hit the brake, but rather than me keeping my feet on the brake, I hit the gas. We headed straight toward the houses that stood in front of us, but before the car could cross the curb and onto the sidewalk, the car came to a complete stop.

I looked over at my teacher that's when I realized he had pressed down on the emergency brakes that was underneath the dashboard on passenger side. He looked at me with disgust on his face.

"Get Out!" he screamed. He scared me so badly that I immediately got out of the car and I begin to walk back up the hill toward the school.

"Where you're going?!" he asked. Get back here and get in the back sit.

I got back in the car while the other student who drove wonderfully back to the school, which I honestly didn't know for sure if I passed his class or not but it he made me even more scared. Even my mother and father tried to teach me how to drive—no luck.

My father taught my oldest sister how to drive before we moved to Montgomery. My little sister and brother learned from some of their friends, but I was the only person in our house that didn't know how to drive. I would normally sit on the passenger side while one of my siblings drove me where I needed to go, or I'd hang out with them while they drove around in my mother's car to run errands for her.

I could remember one night that it was very late—around midnight. My mother was asleep, and my little sister and I got our hands on her keys so that we could drive around Montgomery because we were so bored. We drove around to most of the clubs to see if we saw any of our friends hanging out in the parking lots at the Krystal restaurant

My sister and I didn't care about the consequences that might be waiting for us once we got home; we were trying to find something to do that night. Once my sister drove back onto McElvy Street, she turned off the headlight as we slowly drove down the hill toward our house. Once we got down the hill, we noticed a light beaming from the center of our house, and as we got closer, we noticed our mother was standing in the door with rollers in her hair. "It's Momma!" I said. Keep going! She's going to kill us.

As we drove passed our house, we made eye contact with her, as she stood with both of her hands on her hips. We eventually went back home where she punished us for taking her car without letting her know. But as I look back, our mother had her hands full when it came to the four of us but she didn't love us any different, which she taught us to respect ourselves and others too.

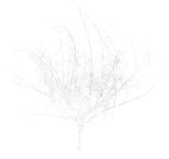

THE FRUSTRATION OF UNDERSTANDING

I was a little upset with my siblings they still haven't gone in to be tested but I didn't say anything. They had there own reason for not going in yet. I knew deep in my heart they will eventually go in, I just didn't know when.

I didn't feel like my normal self. I didn't have any strength. I would just lay there on the sofa and watched television because I was afraid to eat anything because I might throw it back up. And when I did eat, I couldn't taste the food that I was eating.

During that time, while I was at home sick, James was studying for his real estate license. He had failed the first test so he was trying to retake the test. He insisted that I helped him study because he was afraid that he wasn't going to pass. As I lay on the sofa, he sat across from me. I called out questions from his booklet, while he tried to give me the answers to them. I was so weak. I could barely talk or sit up, but not once did he ask me if I was okay. I lay there thinking to myself; *Only God can handle James—in his own way.*

After my second treatment, the bone biopsy showed that I wasn't in remission. A week later, I went back home. I got up mostly every morning and sat or lay on the bathroom floor with a blanket. As I lay across from the toilet, I waited to throw up. It became a normal routine for me after each treatment.

I lay there patiently sometimes, or if I wanted to get it over with, I'd stick the tip of the toothbrush down my throat to get it over with so that I could feel a little better. The taste in my mouth was gone so I had to eat something that was very light on my stomach. I knew if I tried to eat something heavy it didn't stay down long.

Most mornings, I'd sit on the bathroom floor and listen to the radio, but one particular morning as I sat on the floor, I heard them talking about this ex professional football player whose little daughter was diagnosed with Leukemia. They was asking people to come out on Saturday at the Texas Stadium in Irving because they was holding a blood drive to see if they could find a donor for his daughter.

As I sat there, I thought *that was sort of strange. I had seen him and his wife with their daughter on television one night.* They were interviewed by a news anchor because they were so desperate to find a donor to save their daughter's life. After that day, I sat or lay on the bathroom floor every morning waiting to throw up and to see if the radio station would give an update about the little girl.

I thought since they was having this blood drive at Texas Stadium, maybe James would be willing to go down to get himself tested also. Later that day, he walked into the apartment and was about to walk to his room. He walked down the hallway toward his room, but I stopped him. I needed to talk to him, but I didn't want to go into the bedroom that I had once shared with him.

"James," I said.

"Yea," he said.

"Why you haven't gone in to be tested to see if you'll be a match for me?" I asked. Are you scared?

As he stood in the entry of his bedroom, he never turned around to face me. He walked into his room.

"No," he said. I'm not scared, DD.

DETERMINATION

"James I can respect you if you're afraid, but I don't understand why you haven't gone in yet if you said that you loved me?" I asked. *James? Why haven't you gone in to be tested yet?*

"I am, DD."

"But why you haven't gone before now?" *Are you scared?* He stood next to the door but he never turned around to look at me to give me any kind of eye contact because he just kept his back to me.

"DD, I've been very busy," he said.

"Well they're having a blood drive at Texas Stadium for this little child next Saturday maybe you can go in then?" I said.

"Okay," he said. *I can do that.*

He walked into his room and closed the door. I went back into the living room, and I sat there thinking about how I asked God to show me if this was the right man for me. James had told me once that he thought that I deserved someone better than him. I was beginning to think that he was right. *I do deserve better.*

Several days later, I knocked on the bedroom door. I haven't heard anything from James since we talked about him going to the blood drive that coming Saturday. "Yea," he said. He didn't get up to open the door. So I stood there talking to him through the closed door. "James?"

"Yea," he answered.

"Are you still going to Texas Stadium on Saturday?" I asked.

"Yea, I told you I was."

"Will you let me know how it went?

"Yea, DD," he said.

I walked away not being able to understanding why he didn't care that much about saving a person's life. I thought to myself, *if he was in the same predicament I would've gone in immediately because I loved him. Even if I didn't have the knowledge that I have now and he was a total stranger, I would've went in if it was going to save a life.* But that question came back up again, *Does he really love me?*

That Saturday I sat waiting on him to come through the front door so that I could ask him, "Did a lot of people turned out to save this little girl's life?" I prayed that enough people were willing to show up for this little girl. When he finally came home from the blood drive he walked straight passed me while without saying a word.

I got up and I followed behind him. "James?" I said. He wouldn't turn around.

"How did it go?" I asked. Was there a lot people?

"It was very little," he said.

"Very—little? Why?" I asked.

"I don't know, DD."

I turned around and went back to the living room, and I sat there thinking to myself. *This poor baby has been stricken with a disease that she didn't have any control over. She didn't understand why this has happen to her.*

I was very angry, and I started asking myself, *Why was there not enough African American willing to save more lives? Something like this is life threatening. Wouldn't they want to have the same options, that maybe they had a better chance of finding someone with same blood proteins as their blood and maybe the same DNA too? Why are they not willing to save a life? I don't understand.*

At the same time, I began thinking about my own family, again. I couldn't understand why it was taking my own sibling so long to go in to be tested. I called them to ask them if they was still going in to one of the clinic in their area to see if they was a match, but they gave me a lot of excuses that went on for several months. I began to wonder did they not care about their own sister or were they afraid, too? Why weren't my white friends afraid to take a chance to save my life?

I grew up in a Baptist church, and I was taught to put a lot of my faith and fears in God's hands. Why should it be different for others? I guess they are afraid to give someone else a better chances to live because of their own fears, but God gave us so much knowledge by giving our doctors the skills they needed to save lives.

What was wrong with this picture? I guess only God could answer those questions. I was so angry and disappointed that day. But I guess if I was in their shoes and I didn't have the knowledge or I didn't understand how serious this disease was, maybe I would probably be ignorant about Leukemia too. I knew I couldn't look down on them but I had to accept that they just didn't realize how sick I was or maybe they were afraid.

I was afraid of a lot thing too. I tried to block them off by ignoring the situation at hand. I loved my family but I also had a way of pushing people away. With my life on the line, I thought a lot. I would normally lie on the sofa where I thought about my family especially my father.

After our parents' divorces, we used to visit our father doing the summer. He eventually moved to Eutaw so that he was closer to his job. While we were in Eutaw, my oldest sister drove us to Forkland a lot to visit with our grandmother while our father was at work. They moved our grandmother from her old house once our grandfather died and they built her a new house next to our cousins. It was strange because things had changed so much when we left Marengo County.

Our cousins were older now, and they were attending college at the University of Alabama in Tuscaloosa. I felt a deep loss and such loneliness when we were there. I missed the time we spent together when we were younger and the bond that we used to have. We had all grown up, and we all went our separate ways, and now the great times we had together are in the past.

Whenever we came to visit our grandmother, she was always sitting by the window in her living room in her new home as we walked inside. She had so many pictures of all her grandchildren, which were a lot. I've forgot how many grandchildren or cousins I had, but she had pictures on the mantles, on the walls in the living room, and especially throughout the hallway.

We use to sit and talk with our grandmother for a while before we headed back to Eutaw so that my sister could pick up our father from work. Sometimes my father would go back to my grandmother's house to cut her grass or sometime feed the dogs from the food from the cafeteria. Afterward he would sit awhile and talk with our grandmother, before we headed back home to Eutaw.

The very last time we visited our father my mother drove me, including my little sister and brother, to Forkland for a family reunion we were having that summer. I was very excited because I wanted to see my cousins, but as usual, some of them weren't there because they were at college or working, but I was fortunate to get a chance to see one of my cousins and other family members.

During our visit, things between my mother and I were different. We weren't getting alone at all. We were at each other's throat for small and irrelevant things that weren't that important. After the family reunion, my mother drove us to our father's house to drop us off to spend a month with our father for the summer. Once we arrived at his house, my mother told him how she was having such a difficult time with me and she thought it would be best that I lived with him for now.

I sat on the sofa listening to their discussion, and I was so scared what my father was going to think or say that I sat very quietly. She told him about my attitude and how she couldn't deal with me anymore. My father sat in his recliner and he didn't say a word as he listens to everything my mother had to say.

"Dee is growing up. You have to realize that when you have two women in the same house there's going to be confusion," he said. I sat listening and soon I realized that he didn't take either side. He was a being realistic with both of us when it came to a mother and daughter's relationship. I guess by my father dealing with students

Determination

at his high school and their parent he probably knew how to deal with this type of situations.

We had chores while staying with him, too. We had to take turns washing dishes and keeping the house cleaned while our father was at work. At this time, he was working two jobs. He was still teaching at the high school, but he was also working part time at a dog track in Tuscaloosa, Alabama.

He still got up early on Saturday morning to cut his lawn and trimmed the scrubs. When he wasn't working his second job, he would come home and started dinner before taking a cold shower, which was something he did during the hot summer days. After showering, he sat in his black recliner smoking his Winston's cigarette, relaxing as he watched the news while the food simmered on the stove as we sat the table for dinner.

Some nights, our father cooked outside on his barbecue grill or he cook deer for dinner. It has been time after we left our grandmother's house heading back to Eutaw our father would stop by this very small house that stood near Highway 43. We would get out our father's car and walk through the open door where I saw a man sitting on a bar stool near a very large glass tank that was in the middle of the room.

I noticed there was dirty smoky water inside of this glass tank, but as I got closer, I realized there were live catfish swimming around in there. My father walked up to the man and he asked him to pick out several catfishes. I watched as the man pulled our several of the fishes from the tank and cleaned them while we waited. Once we were home, my father fried the catfish, and we ate it with steamed vegetables and rice. My father was a good cook.

As we sat at the table, we held our heads down while our father led with the blessing, which was still one of his family traditions. After dinner, we remove the dishes from the table and cleaned the top of the glass table so that the four of us could play spades until we were too tired to play anymore.

Our last week we spent with our father, I remember one Saturday when our father had my little sister and brother outside racking and piling grass and they put them in plastic bags while he cut his yard. He told me to stay inside to clean up while they stayed outside in the hot sun doing chores in the yard. I felt guilty, but my father insisted on me staying inside where it was cooler.

In a way I kind a felt that my father was making up for what had happen in the past when I was younger. I wasn't sure but it felt that way because I noticed he didn't take sides with my mother. I learned so much about my father while I was there that summer. My father was a very compassionate and caring person. His friends and neighbors spoke very highly of him when they came over to play cards with us sometimes. While we were there, I remember one his students told us how our father sometime loan his car—a black Cadillac—to his students so they could attend their proms.

While I was there, I stopped being afraid of him. I learned to have so much respect for him. I realized that he wanted us to grow up with a lot of moral values and to have respect for ourselves and others and to also work for what we really wanted out of life.

Before he took us back to Montgomery that same week, he called me back to his bedroom because he wanted to talk to me alone. I followed him into his extra bedroom as he went into the top dresser drawer and pulled out a legal size document.

"Here," he said. Take this and hold on to this.

What is this, Daddy? I asked.

"Dee, I prepared a will for you guys in case I might die."

"But—, Daddy."

"I want you to take this and hold on to it, okay?" I didn't know what to say as we walked into the hallway I looked down at my father's will because I was so shock that he would even think that he was going to die.

"But, Daddy, you're not going to die," I said.

"Dee, I have been in and out of the hospital because I have a bad heart," he said.

"But—Daddy," I said.

"I have glaucoma and I'm losing my eyesight. I need you to hold on to this Will, okay?" he said.

"Okay."

I stood in the hallway thinking that it was no way my father was going to die. He wasn't going anywhere anytime soon. He was going to be around for a very long time. I didn't think anything else of his will, but I was so glad that he trusted me enough to personally share something as private as his will with me.

As my father was driving us back to Montgomery, we had to pass through Demopolis; he decided that he wanted to stop to visit Bertha James in our old community. He told us that she was very sick, and they didn't know how long she had to live. He wanted us to give our respects to her.

As we walked into her house, we all sat in the living room while our father went into her bedroom alone as they closed her door as we waited. He opened the door.

"Dee?" He said.

"Yea," I said.

"She wants to see you." My father said.

"Me?" I pointed at myself.

"Yes. They said that she has been calling your name a lot. Come on," he said.

I got up and I walked toward her room with my father. I was six years old when we left the community, and I hadn't seen her since and she was on her dying bed asking for me. *Me?* I thought. I walked into her room slowly, as my father walked behind me.

The room was very dark as I noticed the curtains were closed. As I got closer to her bed, I noticed she was laying there so peaceful, and I could still see the same beautiful face that was there eleven years ago.

"Bertha, Dee is here." This woman said.

"Dee?" she said.

"Hi, Miss Bertha James," I said. She stared at the ceiling not making any eye contact with me. I looked back at my father trying to figure out what I should do or what should I say.

We eventually left, but as my father drove off, I stared back at the house we use to live in and her house promising that I would never forget her, she was really a beautiful woman who I will always love.

Our father drove us back home to Montgomery, where we said our good-byes to him. I stood on the front porch as I watched my father drive down McElvy feeling such a loneliness for him because he was going back home alone. I thought maybe I should've stayed with him so that he wouldn't be alone.

I realize that day we would never be a family again and that I loved my father. We really didn't take the time to understand him and what he might be going through, but the month that I spent with him I put away a lot of pain that I carried around. I began to feel his pain. He was all alone without us.

After graduating from high school in 1983, I decided to take a year off before I decided to attend Alabama State University, which was my father's alumna. The university was located in my hometown, so I was able to live at home with my family. I was admitted in September, of 1984.

I lived five miles away from the college campus, and I got up around five o'clock in the morning so that I had enough time to eat breakfast, get dress, and walk a couple of blocks down the street from our house to the bus stop. I then caught the bus that took me downtown, where I had to transfer to another bus that dropped me off right in front of the campus for my first class, Sociology, which started at eight thirty in the morning.

After my classes, I walked across campus to their library, where I would sit in one of the vacant booth on the second floor to study.

Determination

After a month in college, I eventually begin to make friends while I studied in the library. Soon, I became friends with Naomi. We eventually began to meet after our classes. We became very fast friends because we had so much in common.

It was as if we were sisters. We had a lot of respect for one another because we didn't have to be around each other every day for us to know that we were good friends. But when we were together, we had so much fun because we were able to laugh at each other's faults without tearing each other friendship apart. I admired her so much, because she was a type of person who wasn't judgmental toward others.

Naomi was pretty and very tall. I admired and was also very jealous how long her legs were. Naomi and I lived a couple of miles from each other, but that didn't stop us from seeing each other whenever we wanted to. We would meet each other half way. I spent a lot of my time with her family. She lived with her grandmother, which I grew to idolize and admired so much because she was so sweet and cared about everyone.

Naomi's family always made me feel as if I was part of their family. I enjoyed and admired the bond they had for one another. I felt it was a blessing that I met Naomi. It wasn't that I didn't have the same bond with my family, but I enjoyed the closeness they had with one another. I felt at home and drawn to her family. I wanted to be a part of their lives.

I loved Naomi's grandmother. Mrs. Richards was the warmest, most loving and compassionate person I ever met in my life. I knew exactly where I stood with her. She was very honest about how she felt about everyone, but there was sweetness about everything that she said or did that I loved and respected about her so much. She had a lot of wisdom, but she was very caution and very protective when it came to Naomi, especially when it came to whom she was hanging out with. She raised Naomi, and Naomi called her Momma.

Mrs. Richards told me once that she thought that either Naomi was going to follow my ways or I was going to follow Naomi's way. She noticed that Naomi was following my way that's why she let her and I hang out together. That said a lot about me and what she thought of me too which mean a lot to me when it was coming from her.

During the fall semester, I met Lauren's father while I was studying in the campus library after my classes. When I first saw him, I thought he was very nice person and very handsome. He stood six feet tall, very clean cut, and medium size build.

During the summer, we spent a lot of time together, especially with my family. I thought that everyone liked him whenever he came over to visits. I thought that he was very polite and nice to everyone, but after he left one evening, my mother called me into her room and she suggested that I not see him anymore and that he wasn't welcome at her home anymore.

I was shocked as to why she would think this way about him. I thought *that he didn't do anything wrong. He didn't come off rude or disrespectful in any kind of way while he was at our home.* At the time, I couldn't understand where she was getting all this from, but I guess it was that mother's instinct. I guess it was something she heard, but it was obvious she saw something that she didn't like about him. I couldn't do anything but to abide by her wishes.

Even though Joseph wasn't invited to my house, I didn't take my mother's advice, and I began to see more of him on campus. I eventually became pregnant. I then decided to drop out of college so that I could have my child. Once I broke the news to Joseph that I was pregnant, he wasn't excited about the news, but we became very distant.

I didn't care. This baby was part of me, and I would be able to share some of the loneliness I felt inside. I had so much love to give, and I just wanted to share it with my child so that I could give it the same moral values that my parents tried installed in us. During my pregnancy, I applied for government assistant to help with prenatal care for the birth of my child.

At first, I was afraid to break the news to my father that I was pregnant because he tried so hard for us to have moral values. I thought about it hard before I put the letter in the mailbox because I didn't know what to expect or what he was probably going to think.

I wasn't sure if he would be disappointed in me. He wrote me back stating that he wasn't aware that I was pregnant until I wrote him about it. He told me to keep my head up and that I should go back to college to further my education for my child and myself.

While I was pregnant, I wasn't getting alone with my mother most of the times, so to avoid any confrontations with her, I mostly stayed at Naomi's house because she was the only friend that I had who didn't care about my appearances or how big I was getting whenever we was in the public.

Whenever I would spend the night at her house, we used to sleep until Mrs. Richards left for work in the morning, and then we would get up to clean the house. I love Mrs. Richards so much that I got to the point that all I wanted to do was sit and talk with her more than Naomi because I learned so much from her. She was so precious to my heart because she's a genuine person. I became so attached to her that I began to learn a lot of her wisdom and her spiritual belief in God.

I had so much fun staying with Naomi's family during my pregnancy. We would all sit around and laughed and teased one another. While I was there, I used to watch Mrs. Richards as she baked cakes for her friends for special events which me and Naomi would wash the dishes afterward as I licked the cake mix from the bowls.

When Mrs. Richards had club meetings at her house, Naomi and I would clean the house thoroughly before she came home from work so that way she didn't have to worry about the house. We would sit around later after her members have left and eat what was left over. I ate a lot whenever I was there at Naomi's house. Mrs. Richards was a wonderful cook and I loved her homemade soup!

When I was at home, I slept a lot, or if I were bored, I would sit on the floor and pull my child's little t-shirts and cloth dampers out of the dresser drawer to smell and feel the softness of them. At the time, I wasn't sure if I was going to have a boy or a girl, but I was praying that God blessed me with a little girl. I asked my mother one day, as we stood on the front porch talking, if it was okay if I could name my daughter after my sister who died before I was born. My mother thought that would be great.

Lauren was eight pounds and four ounces when she was born. As I held my child, I realized that she looked so much like my mother. I thanked God for blessing me with a beautiful little girl I cradled in my arms. My mother was so proud of her first granddaughter; she took Lauren around to all of her friends to show her off.

Once we were settled in at home, I didn't know how to handle my newborn child. When she cried late at the night, I couldn't figure out why she cried so much. She was dry and bottle-fed. It didn't make any sense to me why she would cry. My mother came in sometimes late at night to help me calm her down, even though she had to go to work the next day. I was very thankful, but I knew I had to be responsible for Lauren because I made this decision to have her.

I didn't see Joseph during and after my pregnancy. It took me some time, but I realized my mother was right when it came to him. It was obvious that she saw the bad in him before I did. Even though he wasn't there during my pregnancy, I still wanted my daughter to have a relationship with her father because I missed not having the same relationship with my father, and I didn't want to cheat Lauren in that way.

Once he saw his daughter, he was very excited. He came over a lot to spend time with her or he'd pick her up so that he could spend

DETERMINATION

quality time with her. I was proud that he was willing to put that time in with her so that they could build a bond with one another.

Eventually, I received calls from Joseph's mother who asked if I was willing to travel to Florida for a visit. I was fine with that. I wanted to meet her because Joseph thought so highly of her. Plus I wanted her to see her granddaughter. My mother was totally against the hold thing, but I didn't want to listen to her because I wanted Lauren to have a relationship with both families.

I took the Greyhound bus to Tampa, Florida, ten hours drive, which I thought was the longest trip that anyone could ever image. Once we arrived at the bus station, I was greeted by Joseph's mother before we could actually get off the bus.

I knew right off who she was when she walked up to us because Joseph looked just like her. She walked through the isles with a big smile on her face as she greeted us.

"Hi!' she said. How you're doing?

"I'm fine," I said.

"I'm Joseph's mother." It's nice meeting you.

"It's nice meeting you too," I said.

"I want you to know right off that I want to see the baby not you," she said.

I sat there sort of shocked and unsure how I should take that comment. I thought to myself, *Why would she say something like that to me after we road this bus for hours so that she could see her granddaughter? She never met me in her life not until now why would she say that to me?*

I didn't say anything. I sat with Lauren in my arms and just smiled I couldn't turn back. I didn't have the money to buy another ticket. I was too far away from home to even ask my family to come and get me, which I doubt they would have after my mother told me not to go. So instead, we got off the bus; the entire time I thought that my mother's intuition was right again.

131

The trip went very well even after the comment Mrs. Scott made to me. I got a chance to meet Joseph's family, who were very nice to me while I was there. I learned that Joseph was Mrs. Scott favorite son out of the other three children she had. I also gained a clearer understanding that they had a very strong family bond.

Once I made it back home, Mrs. Scott started sending large boxes of things for Lauren. I was very grateful because I knew I couldn't afford such beautiful dresses, toys, and a lot of necessities that she needed. Joseph would sometimes come over to visit Lauren. After his visits, my mother and I would get into arguments about him. I didn't want to hear what she had to say because I still thought I was in love, and he was also the father of my child.

One day after he came and left, he walked out the front door while my mother was sitting in the living room with her company. She excused herself and walked back to my room as we stood in the hallway. I could tell she was mad.

"Dee, wake up!" she said.

"What? What are you talking about, Momma?" I asked.

"You're living in a glass with blinders on where you're not being real to yourself!"

"Momma, he didn't do anything but come over to see his daughter."

"He's no good and you need to wake up!"

She walked back up front where her company was sitting in the living room, and we didn't speak for a while because I was so angry with her. I knew he wasn't there for me while I was pregnant, but I thought that maybe he was afraid of the responsibility of having a child because we both were young at the time.

What really woke me up when I took Joseph to Mrs. Richard's house so that she could actually see Lauren for the first time? Joseph came off very rude and disrespectful when he spoke to Mrs. Richards. *How dare he talk to her that way?* I thought.

Mrs. Richards sat there that day, and she didn't say anything rude about his attitude. I was so embarrassed, and I could see the disappointment and her expression on her face that she didn't care that much of him.

In that moment, I began to observe him even more and began to see what my mother had tried so hard to make me see. As I sat there, something came over me. I looked over at him as he kissed Lauren on the jaw. Suddenly, the blinders came off.

I saw for the first time the arrogant and disrespectful ways that he had toward others. I began to dislike what I saw in him, but it was too late. Reality had kicked in. I knew I had to deal with this man as the father of my child for the rest of my life but I wasn't going to rely on him.

I applied for welfare for Lauren and myself. I took the transit bus to the Welfare office with my child in my arm. We sat waiting until my number was called to meet with my social worker. Once I was called, my social worker she asked me a lot questions to see if I was qualified for their assistants. She went through all the requirements and procedures with me and what I had to do to get qualified for government assistant. As I sat there listening to her, I realized then that I wanted more then this for my child and myself.

I didn't want to rely on the government and their stipulations. I knew I had to take care of my child myself rather than relying on assistants. It wasn't about me anymore; it was about my newborn child. I had to put Lauren first now. I thought about what my father said to me in his letter. "Keep your head up and go back to college," he said. Those words stayed with me, and I decided to go back to college so that I could further my career. I knew I had a responsibility that was relying on me.

MY OWN FEARS AND TRUST ISSUES

Fall of 1986, I went back to college, and I start looking for a job. I filled out a lot of applications at various retail stores, and I was able to find employment at a shopping store, Gaylord's, that was on West South Boulevard. When it was time for me to go to work, I had to take a cab because there weren't any buses that ran on this particular freeway.

While I worked at Gaylord, I did whatever they asked of me. I worked mostly on the floors straightening up items on the shelves or helping the cashiers ring up merchandise. I was willing to work hard to for an opportunity to get the experience I needed to further my career and to have my own finances so that I could raise my daughter.

When I went back to college, it was very difficult for me because this time I had a daughter. When I woke up at five o'clock in the morning this time, I had to get myself *and Lauren* dressed so that I could drop her off at the babysitter before I took the bus to Alabama State University.

Every morning, I put her in her stroller and wrapped her in two or three blankets so that she was warm before I begin to walk five blocks to the babysitter's house. I would be pressing for time to catch my bus to school after I dropped her off. One morning, as

I was walking down McElvy Street with Lauren in her stroller, a woman stopped her car in the middle of the road. She rolled her window down.

"Baby, where you're going with that baby in this damp air?" she asked.

"I'm about to drop her off at the babysitter before I go to school," I said.

"I'll drop you off, get in," she said. It's too cold for your baby to be out in this damp air.

It took me a while, but we got into her car, and she dropped us off that morning. I kept dropping her off at the daycare before I head to school. This went on for a couple of months until my little sister decide to watch her for me.

After the bus dropped me off on campus, I headed to my first class—Art Appreciation, which I had failed the first time when I attended the past year. I decided to take the class over because at first I thought we were going to learn how to paint on canvas and do sculpture, but this class wasn't that at all! It was about appreciating famous art and artists.

At first, I wasn't as serious about my education, but all that had changed because I had a good reason to get a good education—so that I could fulfill my dreams and hopefully give my child a better chances in life so that she could be able dream and hope to accomplish her own dreams too.

In my Art Appreciation class, there was a very handsome guy who sat in front of me in class who fell asleep a lot. Whenever the teacher called on him to answer a question, he always knew the answers or he'd talk around the subject as if he knew the answers. The teacher fell for it each time.

I saw him a lot on campus, and we always smiled or say hello to each other. He came up to me one day as I waited for the bus to come. He introduced himself to me. His name was Raymond. He was twenty years old. He was from Chicago, Illinois. He was at least five foot eleven. He had a light brown complexion and was very clean cut. He was physically fit, but what really made me like him even more was that he had such a beautiful smile. We soon started hanging out.

After our classes was over, he took me home, and we would sometime study together. What I really admired about him was that he knew what he wanted out of life, and he was very determined to reach those goals. And here I was still trying to figure out what I wanted to do with myself.

I changed jobs and started working in the mall at the 5-7-9 Store, which was a good thing because once I got out of school I took the bus to work rather than taking a cab to work. The bus dropped me off right in front of the mall. If I had to work until the store closed, I was able to catch the bus back home or Raymond or my family would pick me up from work.

There wasn't a day that I didn't enjoy being in Raymond's presence because he had so much respect for me and my family. Whenever he came over to my house to study, I knew he came over to spend quality time with me, and my mother really liked him—so did Mrs. Richards, which was a plus.

Raymond drove a dark blue and tan topped Camero. He actually had a television inside of the dashboard. I was amazed that he would actually have a small television in his car (this was back in the mid eighties). He would sometime take me and Lauren out to dinner and a movie, but after each date, he always drove the long way home so that we could spend time together, while Lauren slept in her car seat.

One night after I got off work, I walked into my room, where he surprised me with a candle light dinner. He had to taken one of our wooden round tables and covered it with a white sheet with candles and food he ordered from a local restaurant. I was so shocked that I didn't know what to say or how to act. I wasn't use to something like this, and I fell in love with him because he did things unexpected for me and he was so romantic that all he wanted to do was to see me happy.

I was enjoying every minute we spent together. He was the first man who showed me how a woman should be treated. I also knew he cared a lot about me. Because when I invited him to my sister friend's wedding, he didn't hesitate at all. Some men would have been too afraid to go to wedding with unmarried women because they felt that they were trying to put ideas in their heads about marriage. He didn't care, and we had a wonderful time together.

We simply enjoyed each other's company. It was so special because we didn't think about calling ourselves a couple—not until one autumn day when he took me home after school. We had walked up the street trying to find my sister who was babysitting for me at the time.

As we walked up the street to the last house that was on McElvy Street, where I knew my sister usually hung out though out the day, I noticed she was there. As we walk up the steps toward the house, a little boy came running out the house and he grabbed my hand.

"Are you boyfriend and girlfriend?" he asked. We looked at each other and smiled, but I knew he only was repeating what my sister was saying.

"Yes," he said.

My daughter was couple of months old when I first met Raymond. He wasn't bothered that I had a child, and he included her in everything that we did together. He had grown to love my daughter, and I respected him a lot for that. Some men would be too ashamed to be seen in public with someone else's child, but he told me that there was no way that he couldn't love me and not love my daughter too.

Joseph still came by to pick Lauren up, but he never took the initiative to provide for Lauren while he was still attending college at Alabama State University. Even though his mother was still sending boxes of clothes and toys for her, Raymond gave her what she really needed—the love and compassion that a child needed from a father.

There were times when Raymond brought it upon himself to go to Sam's Warehouse, where he purchased large boxes of Gerber baby food and pampers. I was amazed that he stepped up and brought upon himself to do this for a child that he didn't even father.

He would sit and feed Lauren at the kitchen table after giving her a bottle and burp her before he put her down to bed. I was stun when I found out that he knew so much about babies. He sometimes would give her a bath and would lie near her until she fell asleep. It got to the point that he couldn't leave until she fell asleep. Because when he tried to leave, she screamed.

My next-door neighbor Mrs. Reese asked me several time if I was sure Raymond wasn't Lauren's father because they looked so much alike. Raymond wore his haircut very low and Lauren didn't have any hair at the time, and they had same complexion with big ears. I explained to her that I wish he was her father, but unfortunately, I met him after I had her.

My father hasn't seen his granddaughter yet, and Raymond was nice enough to take us down to Eutaw so that my father could meet his granddaughter for the first time. Before we got there, I asked Raymond to take his diamond earring out of his ear because my father didn't believe in men wearing earrings. He respected my wishes and took it out before we got to my father's house.

Once my father saw his granddaughter, he was so proud. I could tell by the expression on his face and how he tried to be gentle with her as he held her. I was so proud, and I could also tell he really liked Raymond.

Later on that night, he invited us to have dinner with him and one of his friends. As he drove us toward Tuscaloosa, Alabama, he made a right turn down a dark and narrow dirt road, where it was pinched black. The only thing I could see that we were in the woods. He drove us down further into the woods, and I saw a little cabin, hidden away from the road.

He parked, and we all got out. As we entered the cabin, it, too, was very dark, but I soon realized, as one of the hostesses greeted us, that we were in a restaurant. We followed the hostess to our table. There were a lot of drippy candles on the tables, which lit the hold restaurant up. It was very nice and cozy.

On the walls, there were many signatures from various people, who had eaten at the restaurant. We sat and talked as we enjoyed our dinner. The food was very good, and I had the best time with my father. As we said our good-byes, I felt sadness.

As Raymond drove us back to Montgomery, I thought about how lonely my father probably was without us. It brought back so many memories. I sat thinking of all of the good times. Those bad times didn't outweigh the good times we had with our father.

The long drives in the country, playing spades as we got to know each other. I remembered how he uses to sit in his recliner watching his favorite television show, *All in Family* episodes, laughing to relieve the stress of his daily life. It's one thing that I did learn from my father that he felt that common senses could take us further in life than being too book-smart. At the time, I was too young to understand what he was trying to say, but eventually, as I got older, I did.

Raymond and I gotten even closer, my family loved him and our friends thought we made a cute couple. I learned so much from him. He showed me how to take care of my body by eating healthy and working out. But I thought, *How long will our relationship last?* Everything was going so well between us but I just didn't trust Joseph. Whenever, he came for Lauren he became was very demanding and very disrespectful whenever he picked her up.

One night, I received a call from Joseph saying that he would like to pick Lauren up so that he could spend some time with her.

I told him I was fine with him picking her up. I was at home alone that night, and once he walked through the door, I could tell he had been drinking. I could smell the liquor on him. "I don't think she should go with you tonight." I said. You've been drinking,"

He didn't saying anything; he simply tried to take her out of my arms. "No." I said. I turned to walk away but he grabbed her out of my arms.

"No!" I screamed. Give her back to me, Joseph.

All of sudden I felt his hand go across my face twice. I have never been slapped before in my life but once he slapped me it felt like a shock of lightening that went across my face so fast that once I realize what had happen that I didn't know how to react. He walked out the front door with Lauren in his arms.

"Stop!" I screamed. Please stop! I grabbed at his arm as I tried to get my daughter back but he kept walking.

"Please." I screamed. I start hitting him in his back hoping he would react but he kept walking toward the car as I stood in the yard crying. I ran back into the house to call the police immediately. Once they arrived, I explained the situation to them, and they took down my report. But as they walked out the front door, my mother greeted them.

"What happen?" she asked.

"Momma, Joseph slapped me across the face." I said.

"What did you do to him?" she asked.

"What?" I said.

"You had to do something to him for him to slap you," she said. I backed up not believing she would even ask me something like that. It was if she didn't care what happen to me because I felt then that she was on Joseph's side.

"Momma, he was drunk when he came over to pick Lauren up and I didn't want him to take her while he was intoxicated." I said. She said nothing. She walked past me to her bedroom while the police stood watching. I was so embarrassed because now they thought that I probably brought this upon myself.

"Ma'am, we're going to go talk with him tonight and make sure he doesn't go anywhere with your child, okay." One of the officers said.

"Thank you," I said. As they closed the door, I stood there in shock, not knowing what to do next. Neither my mother nor Joseph had any respect for me.

The next day my father drove down to visit my brother because he was giving my mother problems. He was a teenager at the time. When he finally arrived at my mother's home, he decided to sit outside on the porch for her to come home from work. While he sat smoking a cigarette, I walked outside, and I told him what had happen the night before.

He didn't say much; he just sat outside on the front porch while we sat in the living room waiting for Joseph to bring Lauren back home. I looked out the window, and we noticed a car pulling up in front of the house. It was Joseph.

As he walked up on the porch, he was carrying Lauren in his arms. He knocked on the front door. I opened the door, and he gave Lauren to me. I grabbed her and closed the door not saying a word to him. He turned to leave, but my father stopped him.

"If you ever touch my child again, I will blow your head off." My father said. Joseph didn't say a thing he just stared at my father, and then he walked back to his car.

Once he opened the car door, he screamed. "Black Power!" he said. As he raised his fist up in the air like a fool.

"We're all brothers!" he screamed. And we're all equal! We watched through the window shaking our heads as we watched him drive off.

I thought to myself, *What was I thinking about? You're a fool, Dee,* I thought. *Now you have to deal with this man for eighteen years of your life.* I was in for a long and dramatic adventure that will go on for probably a long time until I was able to stand up on my own and learn how to defend what I believed in.

"Dee." I heard my father call my name through the window. I walked outside on the porch.

"Sir," I said.

"If he gives you any more problems, let me know," he said.

"Okay." I said.

"He's young and stupid but I'll kill him if he touches you again," he said.

That day I really had a lot of respect for my father. I knew then that he really loved me and my siblings because he wouldn't have drove over two hundred miles if he wasn't concern about my brother too.

That fall Raymond took us to the football classic in Birmingham, Alabama. Raymond also invited us to drive to Selma to visit with his grandparent. They were very nice, and it was evident that they loved their grandson. They always lit up with inspiration whenever he walked into their home, and whenever we came down to visit, they cooked us dinner.

Raymond invited us to Chicago to visit his family, whom he spoke so highly of and wanted me to meet. I was a little nervous because I didn't know what they would think of me, but it was obvious he thought a lot of me to take me home to meet his family. Some men didn't take women home unless they were serious about them.

We took the trip to Chicago in the month of May. Raymond told me the weather in Chicago would be nice and breezy during that time of the year. I never been up north before, and I was so excited. It would be an adventure I would never forget. I thought his entire family was very nice to my daughter and me.

As we drove back to Alabama, it seems like the drive was quicker. It didn't take us that long to get back. We were exhausted from the trip. As the three of us walked into my home, we noticed a very large stuffed animal, at least four feet tall taking up half of living room sofa. I looked at my little sister who was in the kitchen. "What is this?" I asked.

"Joseph's sister sent it down to Lauren," she said.

"It's so big," I said. What can she do with it? I asked.

"I don't know," she said as she walked back to her room.

Raymond sat down with Lauren in his lap as he cried. "DD, I can't compete with them," he said.

"What?" I asked.

"I can't compete with Joseph's family."

"Raymond, what you're giving to my daughter is more than any of these materialist things that they have sent down to her. Raymond you are giving her love, and that's more important in her life than a large stuff animal. She too small to even play or even remember these things as she gets older, but she will remember one thing that is very important—love." I said.

He sat in the chair as he looked over at the stuffed animal, and he shook his head. I couldn't convince him that it didn't matter. He gave Lauren and me a kiss, and he left. I was devastated as I watched him walk out the front door. He has done more for Lauren than Joseph could ever have done.

I knew Lauren wasn't his responsibility, but at the time, he loved my daughter, and he wanted to be a part of her life. However, he was in college and trying to manage his own finances, I felt that if he could do more for us he would have, but he was frustrated that he thought he had to compete for my child's love when it was always there.

I admired and loved him so much, and I thanked God for bringing him into our lives. He gave us unconditionally love, and he was that type of man that any woman would want as their husband. He was so determined to make it on his own rather than relying on others. He wanted to take the long and hard road to success so that he could've appreciated what it took to struggle to accomplish his dreams.

I had hoped that we would have been able to share our accomplishments together. He was a good man, and he was a good father to my child. Loving Lauren wasn't enough for Raymond. It got to the point that he wanted me to stop Lauren's relationship with Joseph's family because there was something about Mrs. Scott that he didn't like. However, I insisted that Lauren needed to be a part of their lives too which didn't sit well with Raymond.

A couple weeks later Raymond told me that his mother purchased him airlines ticket to fly home to Chicago over the weekend, and when he flew back to Alabama, I saw less of him. I was still hoping that nothing would change between us, but it had. I felt that by me letting my daughter have a relationship with her father and his family; it caused a lot of confusion in our relationship.

Raymond was distant with me. I was very confused and didn't know what to think. He wasn't coming over that much, and he wasn't expressing what he actually felt. One day I was in the kitchen while my mother was cooking dinner, while I sat at the table doing my homework.

"Momma," I said.

"Yea," she said.

"One of my friends asked me if I would do a letter to this sorority to see if they would accept my request to be invited to one of their meetings."

"Oh really," she said. You need to do something because Raymond is seeing someone else.

I turned around and just looked at her. I was shocked that she would even think that something was wrong when it came to our relationship. "What? What do you mean, Momma?" I asked. She didn't say anything else.

I sat there stunned that she would've said something like that to me, even though she really didn't get involved in our relationship.

I got up from the kitchen table, grabbed my book, and I went back to my room. I sat there just thinking about what she said about Raymond. I knew she was right about other things too in the past. I wasn't seeing that much of him lately, and it seemed that I was spending a lot of my time with Naomi and her family.

I didn't see that much of him on campus either. If he wasn't working, he was too tired to see us, but I was still hoping that things between us would get better. But I felt deep inside that it was coming to an end. I just didn't know when or where.

IT WAS TIME FOR CHANGE

After my relationship with Raymond was over, I knew I had to leave. It wasn't anything there positive for me to stay in Montgomery but my child. I provided for my daughter but I felt that I had to get away from all the hurt. I wanted to focus on my future even though I was still in love with Raymond.

Once my little sister found employment, I started taking my daughter back to the babysitter in our community. As I dropped her off in the morning, rushing to catch the bus I looked back to wave good-bye. She stood at the glass door screaming not to leave her.

Once I got to the bus stop I stood there thinking *I needed to find me. I just didn't know how at the time.* I had to figure out something, I wanted my independence so that I could have a better life for the both of us. I just needed to have faith and patients in God and myself because I knew he'd eventually bring it to me when he was ready.

Mrs. Scott was sending Lauren boxes of clothes and toys. Joseph took Lauren down to Florida to visit his parents sometime, but it was a control issue they had over me when it came to Lauren. I knew I had to make some changes in my life for the best, I wasn't getting anywhere when it came to respecting me and my role as her mother. Plus, I was constantly getting into arguments with my mother and I knew it couldn't go on for too long.

Eventually, I decided to go off to school somewhere. I knew if I told my mother about the idea she would've insist that I stayed. I wanted to ask her to watch my daughter until I was situated in whatever college I decided to go to but I felt that it would've been too much for her. She already raised us I didn't want to put more on her.

Whenever Mrs. Scott called to check on Lauren, we discussed my concerns about giving her a better chance in life. I told her that I thought about going off to college in another state but I didn't know where yet. We discussed about the idea of her watching Lauren until I was situated once I graduated from college.

Mrs. Scott told me that she had to leave her youngest son with her mother until she graduated college as a registered nurse. I had my doubts because I didn't want to be without my child. "I don't know Mrs. Scott." I said.

"Dee, when I lived in Connecticut, I had to go to school full time so that I could make a better life for my children," she said. My youngest son was still an infant at the time. My mother kept him until I graduated from college.

"Weren't you afraid that he would forget who you were?" I asked. I wouldn't want my child to forget me, Mrs. Scott.

"Dee, a child will never forget his mother," she said. When I got my child, he didn't want to have anything to do with me at first but eventually he got comfortable with me. Eventually I was able to take him home to live with us.

"I don't know," I said. I was concerned that my child would forget me. I didn't know who to trust or rely on. I wanted more for my daughter and myself.

"Mrs. Scott, let me think about this first," I said.

"Dee, Joseph has a responsibility too. We are not only doing this for you but we're also doing this for Joseph. We want the best for Lauren too," she said.

After we spoke on a constant basis, I felt that I could trust her; I thought she understood that I wanted the best for Lauren and myself. She told me that she wanted to see me do something positive for both of our lives. What made me come to the decisions was the fact she was there for me because I was Lauren's mother, which I could respect her for being honest with me.

While on campus, I went to the library to research on various colleges in other states. I read various books and magazines looking for schools. I noticed an ad on the back page of a magazine about this college located in Dallas, Texas. It was a two-year college. I could earn an Associate degree as an executive secretary. They also provided room and board. I thought. *I would have a career sooner than I thought so that I could care for my daughter and myself on my own.* Once accepted I notified Mrs. Scott about the details of the school.

I decided to take Mrs. Scotts offer. When I said my good-byes to my daughter, it was the hardest day of my life. As I sat in the living room holding her tight in my arms while we waited for her father to come, I was so scared she would forget me. She was two and a half years old when her father showed up that day which I knew I would miss some crucial times in her life but I was looking at our future together in the long run.

There was loneliness as they drove off that day. At the time, I felt that it was for the best because I knew I had to get my life in order so that she would have better opportunities that I didn't have. This was my child. We have a bond that would never be taken away from us but I felt guilt for leaving her but I knew within my heart we would be together soon.

Before I left I had to break the news to Mrs. Richards that I was leaving. We became even close after Raymond and I went our separate ways. She was so patient with me throughout that hold ordeal. It got to the point that my friends tuned me out when it came to Raymond. I was constantly talking about Raymond and our break up.

Not Mrs. Richards she listened and gave me so much inspirational outlook about putting my faith in God first. "Only God had control over your life and the relationship you and Raymond shared. DD, you need to take your hands off Raymond and put your faith in God's hand. Let him handle it because if it's meant for you two to be together it will happen," she said.

I said my good-bye to Mrs. Richards that night. As we stood outside of her house, she begged me not to go. "DD, please don't go," she said. "Please, DD."

"I have to Mrs. Richards," I said.

"Please—," she said.

She had the sweetest and soft voice that I felt so bad. I begin to cry. "I'm sorry Mrs. Richards but I just want more for my daughter and me," I said. Once I left her house, I felt a big loss that night because I loved her so much. She was such a strong figure in my life. I learned so much of her wisdom she was willing to share with me.

She was *the* person who knew my heart without me explaining or convincing her. I knew she loved *me*. She and my daughter were two people I was going to miss the most but I knew I couldn't turn back now. I made this decision and I had to follow through for a better me.

Once I said my good-byes to my family, I was on my way to Dallas, Texas by Greyhound bus. I was shock I made such a major move. When the bus driver *finally* arrived in Dallas, I was amazed how big the city was. I always wanted to come to Dallas; I was a big fan of *The Dallas Cowboys.*

Even though I was excited once I arrived, I was still afraid. I got my luggage off the bus; I noticed there were cabs parked in front of the station. I walked out where one of the taxi drivers asked if

I needed a ride to my destination. I provided him the direction to where I needed to go.

I sat in the back of the cab; the driver showed me various places as we entered I-35. I also noticed the meter was going up.

"How far is the apartment complex?" I asked.

"Oh—we'll be there pretty soon," he said.

As I looked through the car window, I thought Dallas was such a beautiful city and it definitely wasn't Alabama. I knew there were more opportunities here for me and I was going to make the best of it. A week after getting situated at my school and apartment, I found employment within a week. I started working at Sears at the Valley View Mall on Preston Road.

I shared an apartment with two roommates. We didn't have a telephone in the apartment. I had to find the closest telephone booth in the area so I walked up toward Webb Chapel Road so I could check on Lauren, but whenever I called, Mrs. Scott was short with me sometimes.

Lauren would always be asleep when I called. As I stood in the telephone booth, I thought, *what did I do? That wasn't a smart decision you made, DD, by leaving Lauren with Mrs. Scott. She told me that she was there for me.* It got to the point that whenever I called she came up with all type of excuses why I couldn't speak with Lauren.

I begin to miss home but I knew I had to stay in school if I wanted to have a better life. Eventually my mother came around because when I left she wasn't too happy. I called home sometime just to let her know that I was doing fine.

"I want you to know that I'm very proud of you," she said. I hope that you make the most of your education."

"I will momma," I said. I promise.

I wrote my father just to let him know that I was attending college in Dallas. He was very proud of me. I eventually sent him a copy of my official transcript showing the grades I made and how my GPA went up to 3.2 during my first semester. I wanted so much to make him proud.

He wrote back telling me how proud he was of me and if I needed anything to let him know. He also told me that grandparents couldn't raise their grandchildren and I should get Lauren back with me once I finished school.

A couple of months in school, I made friends while attending college. A couple of them warned me including my roommates to stay away from one particular girl who too attended the school. They thought she was wild based on their own personal experience. Well, I didn't listen to them. She invited me to go out with her one night. She wanted me to meet some of her guy friends, which I said okay.

Once she picked me up, she drove us to South Dallas to pick up her friends. She told me earlier that these guys attended Texas A. M. They played football. There were articles written about them in various sport magazines because they would have a successful career playing professional football in the NFL.

When she picked them up, they sat in the backseat while we sat up front. She introduces them to me as she drove around for a while going nowhere. Once we got on I-35 one of the guys asked her for her powder compact and a dollar bill. *Why does he need those two things,* I asked myself.

She fumbled through her purse as she kept her eyes on the road. She reached back and gave them what they asked for. I looked at her as I tried to figure out why they would need those things. I looked back at them while they sniffed this white powder up their noses through a rolled up dollar bill.

My mouth was open. I was shocked. I immediately turned around in my seat as I faced the front looking out the window. I'm thinking to myself *what did I get myself into?* As I looked out the passenger rear view mirror, I saw their bodies jerking back and forth for only a second; eventually they tilted their heads back for a while.

I got so scared I looked to see if there was any policeman around. I didn't want to go to jail for being in this car with these guys. As I turned to look at her, she lit a joint. She passed it around to everyone until she came to me. I told her *No*. I looked at her like, *You got to be kidding?* I guess she thought I was a follower. I had my own mind. I wasn't going to do drugs so that I'll be able to fit in with her crowd.

I couldn't do anything but sit and watch them smoke among themselves. Eventually she took them back to their house. She went inside as I waited in the truck. She came running toward the truck.

"Could you do me a favor girl?" she asked.

"What?" I said.

"Could you drive my truck back to your apartment and I'll come by tomorrow morning to pick it up?"

"No," I said. I don't know my way around this city. You need to take me home right now.

I was getting angry and I could tell she was picking that up too. Plus, I didn't say anything else. She went back in their house *while* I waited in the truck. Once she got back into the truck, I could tell she was pissed but I didn't care. I wasn't expecting nothing like this to happen. As she drove me back to my apartment, I thought, *I couldn't wait to tell my roommates they were right and how I had such a hard head.*

"My friends thought that you were a snob," she said. As she drove me, back to my apartment.

"Oh really," I said. Why would they say that?

"I don't know," she said. But they thought you felt that you were better than they were.

"I am," I said. I wasn't going to put that stuff in my nose or my brain.

"What kind of career can they have doing that?" I asked her. I do have options, you know.

She didn't say anything else to me that night and I didn't care at all. I just wanted her to drop me off so I could distance myself from her. The next day as we walked to school that morning, I told my roommates what had happen that following night. They laughed at me.

"I told you, girl. She was out there but I guess you had to find out for yourself," One of them said. At the same time I was proud of myself that I didn't get caught up in that peer pressure where I felt I had to do drug just to fit in or to be accepted by others.

Every morning, I went to school and afterward I went to work which became a normal routine. While at work assisting customers, my manager called me back into the inventory room. *Did I do something wrong? She never had to call me for anything before especially in regards to my job performances. It had to be something serious,* I thought.

"DD, I have some bad new to tell you," she said.

"What?" I said softly.

"I just received a call from your grandmother," she said.

"Yes."

"I'm sorry to tell you but your father just passed away."

"No!" I screamed. No! Oh—god. I started crying as she tried to hold me but I kept pacing the floor. I couldn't believe that my father has died. She tried to calm me down but I was so overwhelmed over the news that I quickly called my grandmother just to confirm that he had passed away.

As I talked with my grandmother, she told me that it was true. I begin to cry. "What you're crying for child?" she asked me.

"My daddy is gone," I said.

"It's no need to cry," she said.

"Okay." I said. We talked for while and hung the phone up. I

DETERMINATION

immediately called my mother. I told her that I would be coming home on the bus.

I called Mrs. Scott to let her know that my father had passed away, that I was headed home, and if there was anyway she would meet me half way so that Lauren could attend her grandfather's funeral.

"No," she said.

I thought to myself, *What! Mrs. Scott has driven down plenty of times to visit her sister in Birmingham per my mother. She had to pass through Montgomery to get to Birmingham because she stopped through Montgomery numerous times to visit with my mother.*

"I can't afford to bring Lauren to you half way," she said.

"But my father just died," I said. I think she needs to be with my family.

"I'm sorry, DD, but I can't," she said.

"Okay." I said. I hung the phone up but I thought it was time for me to get my child.

The next day I caught the first bus back to Montgomery. My mother and brother picked me up. I thought my mother would be happy to see me. It has been almost a year since we saw each other but once I got in the backseat of the car I could tell after we hugged she was very sadden over my father's death.

Not a word said as we headed to Mobile Height. I realized that even though my father abused her in the past she still loved him. My father always hoped for so long that they gotten back together but it never happen.

Later on that day, I asked my mother how our father died. She told me he died from a heart attack. My brother was with him when he passed away. My brother moved to Eutaw to live with our father. While he ran errands for our father, he noticed daddy sitting on the front porch as he tried to catch his breath. My brother immediately took him to the emergency room where they had pronounced he had died.

I was glad that my brother was with him but my father is gone, I felt emptiness. My sibling and I didn't do right by him, honestly. I wanted to make him so proud. I thought he would live for a very long time.

My mother drove us to Forkland where his funeral was held. While my siblings and I waited at our grandmother's house for the limousines, I knew this was the end. I wasn't ever going to see him again. My grandmother didn't attend his funeral. They thought it would be too much for her.

As I sat in her living room waiting she sat by the window looking at our family as they gathered in the yard. The limousine drove up. I knew it was time for us to go. I wanted to cry but I knew my grandmother wasn't going to have none of it.

I became nervous as I slowly walked down the steps and into the limousine with the rest of the family. My sisters and I cried while my brother sat calmly as he looked out the window. I felt he was at peace. I guess we cried a lot because we didn't have closure. I tried to hold on to my composure throughout the funeral but it was no use I cried throughout the services. I guess I wasn't ready to say good-bye, not yet.

After my father's funeral, we arrived back to my grandmother's house she was still seating by the window as we walked in. She saw our expression as we sat down peacefully. I looked over at her and I noticed she was crying. I never saw her cry before. She was always strong but I felt her pain that day.

That was her baby, her youngest son. Even though my father lived 10 miles away from Forkland to Eutaw, he made sure he came by to see by her mostly everyday. I knew how much my father loved my grandmother, it obvious she loved him too.

I went back to Texas. I felt sadden once I made it back to Dallas but my determination was even stronger. I called my mother a couple of months later to check on her when she told me that my grandmother had passed away. I was sad but I knew I needed to get my life together. I promised my father that I would get Lauren with me once I finished college. I knew my father would've wanted that way.

I was in college for a year and a half and I learned a lot. I felt it was time for me to find a better job making more money. I was missing my baby and I wanted her with me. The little money I was making I saved to buy a bus ticket to Florida to check on my daughter and to ensure Mrs. Scott that after I got out of college I was coming back for Lauren.

When Mrs. Scott picked me up, I was so happy to see my daughter. She was really growing up. I was amazed that she didn't forget her mother. Once she saw me, she rushed into my arms. I held her so tight that I didn't want to let her go.

Once we arrived at Mrs. Scott's house, we sat in the living room chair as Lauren kept looking up at me smiling. Mrs. Scott sat on the sofa as she watched me play with Lauren.

"Dee, can you do me a favor?" she asked.

"Sure," I said.

"Can you go outside and walked around toward the back and come back into the house through the back door?" she asked.

"Why?" I asked.

"I want to see how Lauren going to react.

"Oh—okay," I said. I thought to myself *why she wanted me to do that?* I went outside and walked back through the back door. As I walked into the living room, Lauren was standing on Mrs. Scott's sofa looking out the front window pouting as she tried to see if I was gone or not.

As Mrs. Scott looked on, I slowly walked up behind Lauren as she pulled the curtains to the side as she looked through the window. "Hey," I said softly. She turned around and she smiled as she opened her arms for me to pick her up.

Mrs. Scott smiled but I guess she wanted to see if Lauren actually would forget her mother. I was too happy to see her. I just wanted to spend as much time with her before going back to Dallas. That night she slept with me. We lay in the bed facing one another as she smiled at me while she sucks on her pacifier.

I watched her little eyes closed. The next morning, I turned around she was gone. I looked around thinking that maybe she fell out of bed. The bed was so high for her to jump down. I got up and I noticed Mrs. Scott was in the kitchen cooking breakfast.

"Good Morning," I said.

"Good morning," she said.

"Where's Lauren?" I asked.

"Oh, she's still asleep."

"Asleep." Oh—.

"Are you hungry?" she asked.

"Yea I am. Thanks."

"What would you like?"

"Um, I'll have some eggs and bacon," I said.

Later on that evening as I sat on the floor playing with Lauren in their den I knew I needed to get her back with me. She was getting older and I didn't want her to forget her mother. I needed to be a part of her life. Those days I spent rekindling my love with my baby, I hoped that she knew that I loved her so much.

When I got back to Dallas, I went to the college admission office where I spoke to one of the counselor about my situation. I needed to find employment in my field part time. I wanted to get my child back with me. They found me a part time job working downtown at this small company that dealt with roofing contracts.

Eventually, I started working full time. I dropped out of college so that I could save to bring my daughter here to live but I begin to dislike my position and how the president screamed at one of his employer. It made me uncomfortable that it became to be very intimidating whenever he was in the office. I gave my two-week notice.

I decided to move back home. I was missing my family and

DETERMINATION

especially my child. On my last day, the owner's wife walked down with me to say our good-byes. We stood and talked for a while she told me to take a hold of my life. She went on to explain that she made the decision to stay at home and raise their children rather than furthering her own career, which she regretted.

I was sadden after I spoken with her because she was a really a very nice person who I wished I had gotten a chance to know her much better.

Once I got myself situated at home, I spent most of my time next door with Mrs. Reese. My mother and I was always in a confrontation whenever we were in the same room. I would sit with Mrs. Reese as she lay in bed because she was sick a lot lately. She was so motivating. She was giving me encouragement to go back to Texas rather than living my life in Alabama.

"Mrs. Reese, since I've been home I know how it feels to be away from home now. I loved being on my own. I felt good being on my own and not relying on others. I just got to figure out how to get back." I said.

"Dee, you wouldn't be able to grow here," she said.

"I know Mrs. Reese but I don't know how yet," I said.

"God will find away Dee," she said. You just needed to keep your faith in him.

I would check on Mrs. Reese almost every morning. I would cook her breakfast and bring it over to her. One morning when I knocked on her front door the door would usually be unlocked but this time it was locked.

I walked to the side of her house. I knocked on her bedroom window. I called out to her. "Mrs. Reese?" I said.

"Yes," she said.

"Are you okay?"

"I'm fine baby."

"Do you want company today?" I asked.

"No not today," she said.

"Do you want me to fix you some breakfast?"

"No, I'm not feeling good today."

"Okay then I'll check on you tomorrow, okay?"

"Okay."

That day I spent the night at Naomi's house. When I came home the next day, my mother was in the kitchen washing her hair in the sink. As I walked into the side kitchen door, I noticed she was crying.

"Momma what's wrong?" I asked.

"They should have taken her in to the hospital," she cried. I didn't understand who she was talking about as she held her head down in the sink rinsing shampoo from her hair.

"Huh? What wrong?" I asked again.

"Mrs. Reese died today," she said.

"What? But I talked with her yesterday," I said. As I stared at my mother and I looked over at the window of her house, I was too shock to move. I couldn't get Mrs. Reese off my mind. She wanted me to get my child back and move to Dallas. My neighbor drove me to Florida to pick up Lauren.

Once Lauren was home, I went to the unemployment agency. I filled out applications with various companies as I kept searching for employment. I would sometime call and speak with a counselor at the unemployment agency but they didn't have any callbacks about a job openings for me.

I applied with the State. I took their test, which I scored an eighty-six. I thought for sure I would've heard something by now but months had passed but nothing. Living at home wasn't getting any better. It got so bad that I was constantly in my room crying. I felt that I didn't have a say when it came to my own child.

Lauren followed me once to my room after an argument. As I sat crying she walked up to me and she wiped my tears from my face. I smiled as I held her in my arms. I knew my child loved me even though she saw grown adults acting very immature at the time. I knew then that I needed to go back to Dallas but this time I was going to make it work.

I was so desperate to get back to Dallas. Some of my friends in Dallas thought it would be okay to come live with them until I got on my feet. I asked my mother would she watch Lauren until I got myself situated in Dallas, which she agreed. I took my income tax money that year I brought my first airline ticket back to Dallas.

Eventually Lauren was back in Florida with Mrs. Scott. My mother told me that she was unable to find someone to watch her while she worked. My siblings had their own lives, which I understood. She explained to me that I needed to find employment soon because she realized now that Lauren needed to be with me.

I applied and interviewed at various companies but nothing was coming through for me until I answered an ad where they was looking for a clerk at this financial institution in Addison. I was so happy because I could save my money for an apartment.

I found an efficiency apartment at the Spring Meadows Apartment on Spring Valley Road that was a couple of miles from my job, which I had to walk a mile to catch the bus every morning. There was no furniture at the time I slept on the floor. Once my six-month lease was up, I moved into a one-bedroom apartment at the Wind Ridge apartment on North Dallas Parkway.

The apartment was very spacious. I had enough space for Lauren and plus the school buses dropped the children off right in front of the apartment complex. It was much easier and convenient for me to catch the bus to work. I saved enough money to buy a bed and a sectional for my living room.

I knew it was time to get my child back with me because I had a steady income now. I started putting money to the side to purchase round trip airline tickets for my daughter and myself from Florida to Dallas. I called Mrs. Scott telling her of my plans it seems at first that everything was okay.

Eventually she called stating that she had second thought about

Lauren moving back to Dallas. She felt that Lauren should live in Florida with her family. *What?* I thought. I didn't argue with her, I begin to think of ways to get my child back with me. I was shocked she pulled this but it told me that she really didn't have any respect for me or the love I had for my daughter.

When she told me that she was there for me, I felt then that it was all a lie. I was *determined* to get my child with me. I brought bus tickets from Florida through Alabama and Arkansas straight to Texas. I asked her if it was okay that I picked her for a visit with my family in Montgomery, which she thought it was fine.

Once my flight arrived in Tampa she picked me up from the airport. She didn't bring Lauren with her this time. As she drove me to her home, it was very quite. I wasn't going to say anything to piss her off or let on what my plans were.

"I think that Lauren would be better off here with us," she said.
"Why?" I asked.
"All of her friends and family are here," she said.

I didn't say anything. I listen because I had it all planned out. I knew whatever I said didn't matter because she felt that she had that right. I trusted her with her story about her youngest son. *Why did you listen to her?* I thought. *How could I've listen to her when she told me she was reluctant to leaving her child while in college?*

I feared leaving my child behind but she assured and trusted which was a big mistake I made. I couldn't blame her for how she felt for her granddaughter. She loved her and I understood her family was attached too but I wanted my baby. It was my dream and my motivation to take of my child on my own. I felt like a thief who was about to kidnapped their own child. I thought *I didn't know how to stand up for myself.*

I came off very passive and quiet while I was at her house. She took us to the bus station. I thought about how I wasted my money on airline tickets when I had to purchase bus tickets just to get my

DETERMINATION

child. I was making it barely on a fixed income but I didn't care I wanted my child.

When we said our good-byes, we got on the bus headed toward Alabama, but really, we went through Arkansas to Texas. Once I got Lauren situated in our new apartment and enrolled into school I was served a summons to appear in court with Lauren. Mr. and Mrs. Scott filed for full custody.

I begin to freak out. I never had to appear in court in my life especially for something that was my own flesh. I didn't know what to do. When I got to work, I talked with my supervisor. He suggested that I find an attorney. I found an attorney who dealt with family law.

The attorney had a small law firm on Northwest Highway and Hillcrest. After Lauren went off to school, I took the bus to meet with her. I explained the entire situation to her. She stated she would be happy to represent me during the proceedings.

I also explained I didn't have much money. She still was willing to work something out with me. "What do you do for a living?" she asked me.

"I work as a clerk at FDIC," I said.

"Would you be willing to come to my office over the weekend to work to payoff my fees?" she asked.

"Sure." I said.

I showed up at the Dallas District Courthouse with Lauren. I was really nervous as we entered the courthouse. They put Lauren in another room during the hearing. I noticed Mr. and Mrs. Scott and their attorney seating on the opposite side of the room. I didn't make eye contact with them as I sat down with my attorney.

Once the judge came into the room, we stood up until he sat down at his bench. As their attorney stood up to present their cases to the judge, my attorney tried to explained her defense for me. After he heard what both attorneys had to say, he stated to the attorneys that he couldn't hear our cases. If Lauren had lived in the state of Texas within six months, he could've given a judgment.

He suggested that Lauren had to go back to Florida with her grandparents. I had to fight for custody in the state of Florida. I looked at my attorney with tears running down my faces. *I couldn't believe what just happen,* I thought. They took Lauren into custody as I sat in the courtroom shocked over what had happened.

My attorney left for a minute to talk with the judge. I sat in the empty courtroom crying thinking about what sources or funds I needed to find an attorney to represent me in the state of Florida. Eventually, my attorney came back into the room. I followed her into this small library. There were a lot of legal books, she begin to fuddle through as she called various attorneys in Florida trying to find someone who was willing to take my cases.

I couldn't stop crying though. "It's going to be okay. I'll find someone for you," she said. We sat for an hour as she called various attorneys in Florida who lived in the jurisdiction that was located in Mrs. Scott's county. She found an attorney that was willing to assist me after she explained my situation to them.

Six months had passed my attorney in Florida notified me that a trial date was set including a deposition on the same day. I immediately went to my supervisor's office where I explained my situation to him. I asked him for a week off which he agreed.

"How you're getting there?" he asked.

"I'm going by bus," I said.

"I can loan you the money to fly round trip if you like?"

"If you don't mind, I promise I'll pay you back," I said.

"I know you will Deagara," he said.

I told my mother about my trial date. She decided to take off her job to support me while I was there. After my attorney picked me up from the airport, he also picked my mother up from the bus station. He explained what to expect during the deposition that was held the same day.

I found out that there were actually two attorneys, Mr., Mrs. Scott's attorney, and Joseph's attorney. I was surprised. I wasn't aware that he was involved. He lived in California at the time.

As I sat across the table from the Scotts and Joseph's attorneys, I got scared. I tried to talk when they asked me a question but my mouth got so dry that my attorney had to stop the deposition so I could drink a cup of water.

My mother sat next to me. She tried to calm me down. I was a nervous wreck. "Calm down," she whispered in my ear. If I see that you're getting upset I'm going to touch you on your thigh, okay.

"Okay." I said.

As the deposition proceeded, their attorneys went back and forth asking me various questions. I noticed there was a court reporter that sat across the table from the room. As her fingers moved in a fast pace she watched my expression on my faces.

"Ms. Robinson what was your reason for letting the Scotts keep your daughter?" The attorneys asked.

"I wanted a better life for my child." I said. I thought Mrs. Scott was there for me and my daughter. Once I finished college and on my feet, she knew I was coming for my child. I begin to get upset. My mother kicked my leg. I took a deep breath as I sat back.

"Shouldn't your daughter come first?" The attorney asked.

"Yes." I said.

"So why did you wait until now?" he asked.

"Because this is my child and I'm her mother," I said. My mother kicked my leg again. I looked at her because I was really getting angry but I looked at both of their lawyers.

"I'm sorry but I didn't want to rely on welfare to take care of me and my daughter. I went to Texas to better my self and my life so that I could take better care of my child," I said. I looked over at the court reporter as I took a deep breath. She winked at me and smiled while her fingers took down every word I said.

I felt that what I said made a difference because after I looked over at her I begin to relax and I was able to answer all the questions they wanted from me. Later on that evening, I had to appear in court so that the judge could hear my cases. I haven't seen Lauren in awhile which Mrs. Scott stated in her Answers that Lauren didn't know me.

As we walked into the court, Lauren saw me sitting in the booths. She ran up to me and gave me a hug. She also followed me into the courtroom. As she sat in my lap, the Scotts and Joseph's attorneys observed what just happened.

The bailiff asked that Lauren be removed from the courtroom doing the hearing. My attorney asked my mother could she sit with her until the hearing was over. Once the proceeding started, I noticed Lauren at the door peeping through the door window as she tried to see if I was still there. I begin to cry when I saw here.

Once the trial had begun, I couldn't stop crying. I tried but the tears kept falling. The judge stated that he wanted to look over all documents in his chambers before he made his final decision. He suggested visitation for me while I were in Florida but he instructed me that I had to stay in the jurisdiction.

After the trial was over, I went to water cooler for a drink of water. As I walked to the cooler Joseph's attorney appeared. "Excuse me," she said.

"Yes," I said.

"I hope you get your daughter back with you," she said. I was shock because she really gave me a hard time but I knew she was only doing her job.

"Thank you," I said as I walked away.

We mostly stayed at the hotel. We didn't want to take a chance driving into a different county by mistake. I definitely didn't want to lose the custody of my child. The next morning my mother took Lauren back to Mrs. Scott's while I stayed at the hotel. I called for a shuttle to pick me up.

My flight left the following day but I couldn't afford to stay another night at the hotel. Once the shuttle dropped me off at the airport I spent most of the day sitting, walking or standing by the window as I watched the planes lift off into the air as they flew to their destination. Later on that night, I slept in a chair. In the morning, I woke up with a crook in my neck.

Once I was back in Dallas, I thought *Will the judge give me my daughter back to me.* My mother called to inform me I needed to get Lauren. She noticed how out of control and spoiled Lauren was and she felt she needed to be discipline before she got any older.

Within a couple of months, my attorney called me. He informed me that the judge decided to let Lauren live with me. The Scotts will have visitation rights during the summer and every other holiday. Joseph gave up all of visitation to his parent, which was fine with me. It didn't matter to me; I just wanted the opportunity to raise my child.

When Lauren arrived to Dallas, it was an adjustment for her at first. They basically gave her whatever she wanted and I definitely didn't have the finances like they had. During the hearing, the judge set an order that Joseph should pay child support. Once the judge decided to give me full custody of Lauren, Joseph explained that he wasn't going to pay me any child support.

So I provided her the necessities that I thought was most important for her needs. Mrs. Scott sent various boxes of clothes and other items but that wasn't putting food on the table.

I still didn't know how to drive. I took the bus to go to the groceries store and a cab to take the groceries home. I was lucky though because I lived right off of Dallas Parkway and Beltline. The groceries store was a couple blocks away.

During the summer, Lauren spent the summer in Florida. I called shuttle whenever I had to take her to DFW Airport. Lauren was 5 years old now. She was older enough to fly alone with one of the stewardess assistance. I was frustrated taking the shuttle back and forth to home. The driver drove around the airport least four times picking customers before he left the airport.

Whenever it was time to take or pick Lauren up from the airport, she always was the first to get on the plane and the last to get off with the airline stewardess. It seems that every time Lauren spent the summer in Florida she came back twenty pounds fatter. It put me in a bind with the clothes she had at home that couldn't fix her.

We had to wait a couple of months before she was back to her normal sizes. I didn't like seeing my child fluctuate with her weight when she came home. Eventually Lauren became unhappy with her weight. I noticed how she admired other kids who were smaller. I knew I couldn't put a stop to it because there was a court order. I was so hurt. I tried to talk with Mrs. Scott but nothing came of it.

Every summer she came back overweight. She basically let her eat whatever she wanted during her visit. Mrs. Scott didn't let Lauren bring some of her nice clothes home to Texas. But as Lauren was getting older, I knew she was hurting my child and I couldn't stop her.

We eventually moved to Preston del Norte I condominium on Preston Road. We had our own rooms this time. I bought her a bump beds for her room, which I assembled myself. I wanted to surprise her when she came home from the summer. I decorated her room with Aladdin.

When I picked her up from the airport, I waited as the stewardess brought her through the doors. I noticed that she was even heavy than I seen before. She was tanned; her skin was so tight and thick. I didn't say anything I was just glad to see her but she looked unhappy.

"Hello." I said.

"Hello," the stewardess said.

"Are you Lauren's mother?" She asked.

"Yes."

DETERMINATION

"Can I see some type of ID?"

"Sure." I gave her my ID. I looked at Lauren and smiled but she didn't smile back.

"What's wrong?" I asked.

"Nothing," she said.

"Did everything go okay?"

"Yes."

As we went down the elevator, I looked in her eyes. "What wrong?" I asked her again.

"The stewardess asked me why were you're so skinny and I wasn't," she said.

"She shouldn't have said that to you Lauren." I said.

"I'm sorry, Mom," she said. I told my grand-mom not to feed me this way.

"It's okay Lauren but Mrs. Scott knew better though," I said.

"She made me take ex-lax before I came back to Dallas."

"What?! Why did she do that? I asked.

"I don't know," she said.

I took a deep breath but I was angry because she knew what she was doing. She was hurting my daughter. When the shuttle dropped us off, I immediately called Mrs. Scott up long distances. Before she could get a word in, I interrupted her. "Mrs. Scott, why do you feed my child like this? I asked.

"Why!" She screamed. Dee, I don't think it's nothing wrong with her.

"The hell you say!" This is not healthy what you're doing to my child Mrs. Scott. You don't have an excuse for this. Lauren has to walk around for almost 2–3 months before she got back to her normal size. I can't afford to buy her new clothes. You're wrong for this crap!" I said.

I hung the phone up. I was shock that I just did that but I was angry that my child was fluctuated back and forth which wasn't healthy on her heart. At that time, I didn't care if I hurt her feelings.

I was tired of seeing my child coming back twenty pounds every time she came back home. She had to always deal with the hot and sizzling sun throughout the August and September months.

Whenever I called during the summer, they always complimented me on how well manner she was. They felt that I was doing a great job with her but I don't think they realized they were hurting her by over feeding her the way they were. I was really pissed that day.

An hour after our conversation, my mother called. "Hello."

"What's wrong with you?" she asked.

"What?" I asked.

"Why did you cuss that woman out like that, Dee?"

"But Momma—"

"No, Dee, you're wrong and you knew better," she said.

"But, Momma, she feed my child so much she came back so fat."

"So!"

I started to cry because I knew it was no way I could convince my mother because she taught us to respect our elders no matter what. I knew she was right but I just felt that if my child is telling her not to feed her this way then she should've listen to my child but she didn't.

I tried to get this Child Support Agency to help me get Joseph to pay child support. They pressure him; he begins threatening me. One night I received a suspicious phone call on February 10, 1994. "Hello." I said.

"You're going down," he said.

"What?" I asked. Who is this?

"You're going down." As he talked, I realized that it was Joseph.

Joseph? I asked.

"I'm in Dallas and I'm coming to your house and you're going down," he said. I looked at my caller-id and I noticed that he was at the Radisson Hotel. The area code was (214) so he really was in Dallas, Texas.

I started crying. I was really scared. I immediately called the police and they came out to my apartment. I told them about the phone call I just received. They're trying to make him pay child support but he doesn't want to." I said. I don't want it anymore.

"Well ma'am, he doesn't have any choice." The policeman said. We'll go out and talk with him. After that day, I didn't hear anything else from him but I was still scared and I didn't feel secure where I lived. I looked for an apartment further out of Dallas into the Collin County area.

When I turned 26 years old, I learned how to drive at Sears Driving School. I purchased an old Chevy Cavalier from my neighbor. There was no air conditioner or a radio. I use to put my music box in the car to listen to music as I drove to work in the morning but it was getting me from A to B so I was glad I had transportation.

After I bought the car, I found an apartment in Far North Dallas with a security gates and alarm system inside of the apartment. I was still afraid Joseph might do to me harm if I stayed where I lived. On June 2, 1994, I moved to Idlewyld Village apartments on Haverwood Road. I thought the apartment was very large where Lauren and I bedrooms were on opposite side of the apartment.

Every morning I drove Lauren across town to Plano to drop her off at school. I went to work but once I got off work, I rushed to daycare to pick her up before 6 o'clock to avoid a late fee. It became a difficult time for me. They eventually built a school a couple blocks from our apartment. I requested transfer, which was granted. The classes were much smaller. Plus they had after school care on the premises, which was a good thing because they didn't have to transport her to a daycare nearby.

Lauren was still visiting her grandparents doing the summer. When she came back, she was still coming back twenty pounds overweight but I didn't say anything this time. I would sometime let her go down on Thanksgiving or a week after Christmas which wasn't enough time to cause any weight gain but I noticed that whenever she wanted Lauren to come down to visit other than what the court order specified she would send down boxes of her clothes and a check for $25.00.

The child support agency still went after Joseph. He started calling me again making threats. I was frantic after I got off the phone. It has been times I was afraid to sleep at night even though I had an alarm system. One morning his sister called around six o'clock while I was asleep. "Hello." I said.

"Hey, DD, this is Rhonda," she said.

"Hey," I said.

"Did I wake you?" she asked.

"Yes but that's fine," I said. What's wrong?

"Lauren told us that you hog tied her," she said.

"What?!" I asked. I sat up in my bed. She repeated herself.

"Lauren told us that you hog tied her when she did something wrong." I got out of bed and sat on the edge of the bed so I made sure I heard exactly what she just said to me. I asked her to repeat herself again, which she did.

"So you're saying that my child told you that I hog...tied her?" I asked.

"Yes." she said. I stood up. I begin to pace the floor.

"Why would I do that to my own child?"

"I don't know but that's what she said."

I started crying. I walked to the other side of the apartment and went into Lauren's bedroom. I woke her up as I held the cordless phone to my ear.

"Lauren? Lauren, wake up," I said.

"Huh?" she asked.

"Your aunt, Rhonda is on the phone. She told me that you told them that I hog-tied you. Is that true? Did you tell them that?" I asked her.

"I didn't say that momma," she said.

"Okay." I said. Go back to sleep. I walked back to my room.

"She said that she didn't say that Rhonda. Did you hear her?" I asked. My tone changed in my voices.

"Yea, I heard her," she said. I don't know where this is coming from but I'm just going by what she told us.

"Well I don't know where this is coming from either but I wouldn't do that to my child," I said. I hung the phone up. I was up, I couldn't go back to sleep. I felt that they tried to deliberately make it difficult mentally by making prank phone calls or ridiculous accusation.

My job was downsizing. I started putting my resumes out to various companies but I really wanted to work in a law firm. I responded to an ad in the Dallas Morning newspaper that this law firm was looking for several Legal Secretary.

I sent my resume to them and they called me in for an interview at the Centrum Building on Maple Road. I was interviewed by various departments which I thought everyone was very nice and professional toward me but I admired how the exquisite tastes this law firm had. I wanted so bad to work there. I sent a Thank You Letter to the firm within a week they called and offered me a position.

I started working their on November 15, 1994. I begin getting threats from Joseph at my job because they plan to garnish his wages. His threats at my job got so bad that the law firm changed my work number. Eventually I moved up to two flights of stairs in the same apartment where I felt safer. I notified a personal agency to find out the status in getting Joseph to pay child support but I found out later that they took Joseph's income tax but never notified me.

While I was at work, I sat across the hall from various attorneys, which I asked one of them for legal advice because at the time we had pro bono at the law firm. She helped me as much as she could but she suggested I asked the attorney that sat across from my desk.

At first, I thought maybe she was too busy because she was always in her office late at night or doing research and meeting with various plaintiffs. She stepped in and somehow she had the agency to release all of my documents including my agreement I had with them.

She personally called and filed documents in the state of California to start proceeding for Joseph to pay child support. But we had a lot problems, Joseph forged my names to some of the document and sworn to the court that I agreed for lesser amount of child support.

One of the partners and owner of the law firm helped by sending an order to the judge about the stipulation that was in hand but we were stuck which I was very appreciative due to his busy schedule. My friend and attorney did her best, we even had a hearing with his attorney but nothing really got resolved, and I got to the point that I had enough, I decided to let it run it course with the courts.

FACING MY FEARS

I admitted myself back into the hospital around the first month of November to have more chemotherapy, but this time the chemical was blue. The nurse explained to me that I could have problem with light or the sun, so they gave me a pair of shades to wear during the treatment. The nurses darken my room by keeping the curtains closed. I didn't have any side effect after that treatment.

During that week while I was in the hospital, the nurses gave me a surprised birthday party. They all pitched in and bought me a birthday cake, a card, and a beautiful porcelain angel. I was shock and so happy that they cared that much about me. Later on that night, James came up to the hospital to visit me he brought me a birthday card, but after that day, I didn't see or received any calls from James. I didn't care anymore.

After the treatment, Dr. Howard did another bone biopsy, and the test came back that I was still not in remission. I was scared. I didn't know what to expect or what other options my doctor had. He tried to give me encouragement that there might be other options, but I definitely needed a bone marrow transplant to prolong my life.

The hospital was still waiting on my sibling to go in to be tested. I called them again and I talked with my sister, who was waiting on my little brother to go in with her because they decided to go in together. I thought that maybe she was afraid. She had always been afraid of needles.

I had to go in and out of the hospital, including the clinic that was a block away. It became a routine for me. I felt that the fourth floor was like home. I became familiar with the entire nurses shift that I had most contact with. I knew which days they were off and what hours they had on that particular week.

While I was out on disability, I was receiving only seventy percent of my income. I began to realize all the bills were in my name—not even one bill was in James' name. He would write me out a check for half of the utilities. I paid three fourths of the bills because I felt that it was only fair. I had a daughter, and we had to get a separate room for her.

One day I called various companies to tell them that I was going to be late on my bills. When I called the telephone company, I asked them for an extension until next month. I explained my situation to the representative, and she was very nice and understanding. She gave an extension and told me to read Job in the Bible.

"Job?" I asked.

"Yes," she said.

"How do you spell Job?"

"J O B," she said.

"You mean Job, like employment?" I asked.

"Yes," she said. But his name is pronounced differently though.

"Oh...okay." I said.

"Just read about his story and it will give you so much hope and motivation. Okay." She said.

"I'll do that." I said. Thank you so much.

I got off the phone with her, and I, suddenly, remembered speaking to one of my friend's mother. She had told me to read JOB too. *There had to be something with this,* I thought. So that night, I decided to get my Bible out, and I read the scripture about Job.

Determination

I read about Job. He was a noble person, who feared and respected God. He was tested by Satan, the death of his children, losing his wealth but he didn't give up his faith in God by listen to Satan or his friends, which in the end God blessed JOB with even more.

The following day, I periodically checked my temperature to make sure that I wasn't running a fever. When I looked at the thermometer, my temperature was 103 degrees—even after I took Tylenol various times that day. I immediately called my doctor's office, and he instructed me to admit myself back into the hospital.

Once I was admitted, the nurses constantly gave me Tylenol, trying to bring my temperature down. Still, I would wake up with my clothes and sheets all soaked with sweat. My temperature would go down some whenever they gave me Tylenol, but every time they came in to check my blood pressure and temperature, it would back up to 103 degrees. My doctor decided that they needed to do various tests so that they could figure out why my temperature was so high.

I was taken down for a MRI. They put me in this very large and round object, as I lay inside with earphones in my ear she asked me what radio station I would like to listen to. I told her K104. As I lay there and did exactly as instructed, I heard a beating and pounding sound. I didn't move, and I wasn't bothered by the noise. The test came back negative, which was a good thing. But I was still running a high fever for some unknown reason.

They couldn't figure out what was causing my temperature to be so high, but they were still providing me Tylenol. Later on that day or night, I woke up with my clothes and sheets all soaked with sweat again. The medical assistance was coming into my room, constantly changing my sheets and provided me with dry hospital clothes. As I sat in the chair watching them, I kind of felt that they were getting a little frustrated because they was constantly in my room changing my sheets. I was feeling the same way.

I was in the hospital for days as they tried to figure out why my temperature was so high. I was confused and concern as to why they couldn't find out what was wrong with me. One afternoon, there was a knock at the door. I looked up there was lady standing by the foot of my bed that I never met before in my life.

"Hi, remember me?" she asked. I sat up to take a good look at her.

"No." I said. She came up closer so that I can see her.

"I'm one of the ministers for the hospital, and one the nurses are very concern about you because you don't have any family with you during this difficult time. And she was afraid you might be all alone in the hospitals by yourself," she said.

"But I'm not alone." I said. She hesitated.

"Oh?" she asked.

"I'm sorry but when did we met?" I asked. I knew we never met but she introduced herself as if we had spoken before. I sat there trying to figure out which nurse put her up to this, but she never answered my question. She went on to another conversation.

"I have this Bible that I've brought up for you to read. There are some interesting scriptures you might like to read," she said. She handed me the book.

"Oh—thank you. That was nice of you," I said. I looked at the heading of the Bible. *The News Bible, Today's English Version.* I laid the book in my lap as she looked on.

"So where's your family?" she asked.

"They're back in Alabama." I said.

"So there are no ones here with you for moral support?"

"No. But, thank you for being concerned about me, but like I said before I'm not alone because only God has control over my life, and only he can pull me through this situation. But I really appreciate you giving me this book though. I'll read it, but I just ask that you pray for me," I said.

"Well, okay then," she said. I hope you enjoy the book.

"I will and thank you so much." I said.

If she wouldn't came in as if she knew me then I probably

DETERMINATION

would've open up to her. But she didn't know me, so I was sort cautious. After that day, I began to face my own fears head on. The next the doctors wanted to do a lung biopsy so that they could find out why my temperature was still 103.

When they came to my room to take me down for the lung biopsy they begin to roll me out of my room, but before they could get me out the door and into the hallway, one of the nurses stopped them.

"Can you stop for a second, please?" she asked. I want to first give her something to relax her through the procedure. I gradually pulled my head up, sat up on my elbows, and looked at everyone.

"No. As much as I've gone through, I'll be okay but thank you though." I said. I lay back down on the carrier.

When I was in surgery one the doctors, who I thought was hilarious, told me what was about to happen. "We're going to put you to sleep but we first need to spray this in your mouth that's going to numb your mouth so that I can put a tube down your throat so that I can clip a piece your lung for testing," he said.

Those tests came back negative, and my temperature was still high. I was getting frustrated with everyone, including my Dr. Howard because they couldn't tell me what was going on with my body. I got so tired of laying there doing nothing but sleeping a lot and watching television.

I was constantly asking the nurse to give me something to relax me so that it could put me to sleep so that I could forget everything. After a while, it got to the point that I felt I was getting addict to the medication because I was constantly asking them to sedate me.

One night I noticed they kept a needle taped to my hand, I guess to connect an IV for more testing. Whenever the lab technician came in to draw blood, they usually drew blood from my Hickman. I couldn't figure out why this needle was still there. I sat on the edge of the bed and I slowly pulled the tape off to look at the needle. I gradually removed the needle out of my hand, I began to bleed a little, but even after a few minutes, it wouldn't stop. I got so scared that I called one of the nurses into the room.

"Yes," she said.

"I took the needle out of my hand and I'm bleeding and it won't stop, I said. She immediately walked into the room.

"What?" she asked.

"I removed the needle from my hand."

"Why did you do that?" I could tell she was angry. I start crying.

"I'm tired," I said. I'm so tired. Can you stop the bleeding please?

"Why did you do that?"

Another nurses entered the room, the same nurse who came in to change my bandages. Was the nurse who accidentally pulled the bandage off too quickly, I screamed.

"Leave her alone." The second nurse said to the first. She's tired and frustrated.

"I'm so...sorry," I said. As I stood there still trying to stop the bleeding, the other nurse left the room and the second stayed behind to clean and stop my hand from bleeding by putting pressure on it.

That night, I had the upmost respect for her because she didn't chastise me. I felt that she understood why I was so frustrated. But I got to the point that I began to question my doctor because I felt that he wasn't telling me what I needed to know which would have given me a choice to change doctors, but I couldn't. There was something special about him. But I couldn't put my finger on it. I just didn't know what to think anymore.

I asked one of the nurses about Dr. Howard, and she told me that she thought highly of him. He had such a great reputation among the oncologist community. Then she told me something that made realized how stupid I was. She told me that he went in front of his congregation at church, and he asked if they would be willing to get their blood tested just for me. She went on tell to me that his wife and his wife's father went to the clinic to be tested to see if they might be a match.

I thought to myself, *Well, you did it again.* Not only did my mother insult him by saying that he didn't care about African Americans, but I question his capabilities. I was even embarrassed that he was puzzled why it took my sibling so long to get tested. I started questioning his potential. *Stupid me,* I thought to myself.

As I lay there feeling ashamed for the way I treated Dr. Howard, I also wondered what was going on with my body. I heard a child crying down the hallway that went on throughout the night. I slept for a while when I noticed a nurse came into my room to check my blood pressure and temperature.

As I sat up, I could still hear someone crying. "Is that a baby crying?" I asked the nurse. "No, she said. That's a woman crying.

"Oh—," I said.

"The couple that was next door to you when you first came into the hospital for your treatment, her husband has just died," she said.

"The same couple my mother visited? The same husband who wanted to go home to fix his wife's car?" I asked.

"Yes," she said. I took a deep breath. I was shocked.

"Don't you worry; we caught yours in time," she said.

I sat in the bed stunned and ashamed. My mother wanted me to go over to meet them, but I was so stubborn at the time, angry at the world, and feeling sorry for myself. Now I didn't have a face that I could put with this couple—because of my selfishness.

"I'm going to give you something to relax you." The nurse said. I lay there still in shock, just hoping that he would have made it. I tried to put a face or a picture of him in my head by what my mother told me, but I couldn't. I thought, *If only if I went over to his room to meet them when my mother asked me to rather than feeling sorry for myself.*

I still heard her cries throughout the night. I got out of bed and kneeled down on the side of the bed. My knees pressed down on the cold floors. As she cried, I began to pray for her and their family even though I didn't get a chance to meet them, but once the medication took it affect everything went silent.

Days later, as I was watching television, this very tall man came into the room with a wheelchair. "How you're doing?" he asked.

"I'm fine," I said.

"I need to take you down to the first floor so that we could do more tests," he said. I sat up a little.

"You want to me come with you, right now?" I asked.

"Yes," he replied.

I got out of bed, walked over and sat down in the wheelchair. He put a blanket around my lap. It was becoming clear to me that I was beginning to face things in a much calmer way. I wasn't that afraid as I was before. I guess I was beginning to put more faith in God and realize that whatever happened he was going to see me through this.

As we exit the elevator on the first floor, I remembered really quickly how cold it was down here. It brought back memories of when I was first admitted into the hospital. We went down the same long hallway and made a sharp right turn toward a room that was facing us.

I noticed, as he pushed my wheelchair into the room, that there stood in the middle of the room a very large steel table. As he pushed me closer to the table, he pulled up the leg rest. "Could you get on top of the table for me?" he asked. And I need you to lie flat on your back for me also.

"Okay," I said.

I got out of the wheelchair and gradually got on top of the cold table and I laid there wondering what was he about to do? I looked up at the ceiling and I noticed a very large object that stood above me.

"I need you to lie still for me, okay?" he asked.

"Okay," I said.

He reached over me as he pulled this very large device from the ceiling. I lay very still as I watched this machine move across my body as a little green button was flashing. It was making this clicking sound as if it was taking pictures. As I lay there, I was still wondering why my temperature was so high. *Would this help find the problem?* I asked myself.

After the test came back, the doctor finally found out why my temperature was so high. They noticed there was little fluid around one of my lungs. He told me that I had a slight pneumonia. He suggested then that they should start me on Prednisone. *Prednisone?* I asked myself.

Once they prescribed Prednisone, my temperature was back to normal, and I was sent home. I soon noticed my appetite had picked up too. I begin to put on weight, and my face was getting round and very large—to the point that I was unable to recognize myself anymore.

One evening, James asked me if I would like to have dinner with him. I hesitated to go out in public because I was insecure about the way I looked. We went to a restaurant that was on Plano Parkway. As we walked into the restaurant and the hostess sat us, I kept my head down.

As we waited for our food to arrive, we barely said anything to one another, until finally he brought up about our relationship. "DD, I think that I should move into my own place," he said.

"Oh, okay, I said.

"I haven't started looking yet, but I want you to know that I've learned so much from you. I hope that we could still be friends," he said.

I thought to myself, *He already told me that I should have a man with very high potentials than him He thought that he wasn't the one for me. He was right.* I sat there listening to him and was not even bothered that he was moving on. I was more concern about my life and if I was going to live.

Once we finished our meal, we walked back to his car, and we just sat there for a while. "DD, I want you to know that we tried this, but it just didn't work," James said.

"Have you started looking yet?" I asked.

"I'm sorry but for what?" he asked.

"Apartment," I said.

"Oh, no, not yet."

"Oh okay." We were silent for a while.

"James couldn't you've told me this at home rather in the public?" I asked.

"I didn't know how to tell you," he said.

"James, I realized that you're not the person for me. I've asked God to show me and he has. So, I don't have any animosity toward you. I just think that I haven't found the right man yet, but I hope we can be up front and honest with each other until we go our separate ways," I said.

"I agree," he said.

We sat in his car for about an hour talking as we stared outside at the restaurant through the front car window. We never made any eye contact with one another. I was disappointed that he took me out in the public just to tell me that he was moving out. I didn't care anymore; I just hoped he could keep his word as far as being up front because I had already begun to question the person he really was.

"Again, I just want you to know that I appreciate all you've done for me," he said.

"Oh, you're welcome," I said.

"But I need favor from you," he said. I need you to show me how to cook healthy before I moved into my new apartment.

"Oh, okay. I'll be happy to show you," I said.

"Including my resume," he said.

"You're what?" I asked. I tried to help you before, but you told me that your resume was fine. So—why now?

"I need to find a better job," he said. I'm not happy where I'm at.

I didn't say anything. But I thought, *"You know what? I'm going teach him how to cook healthy food. And I'll help him with his resume and let God fight my battles because I wasn't going to cut my blessing even though he didn't care about me being sick.*

The following day after James told me he was moving out, there was a voice message on the answering machine basically stating that he was approved for his new apartment. The woman on the voicemail went into details about the name of the apartment complex, the location, and the apartment number, but again I didn't care.

God had to show me that this man wasn't for me. I realized that he was definitely a liar because he had told me that he hasn't started looking yet. *I thought we said we would be up front until we went our separate ways?* I would've of been understanding if he told me because I knew we needed to be apart from one another.

Now I felt like I couldn't trust him. He had lied because he didn't have anything to lose by telling me the truth. He really didn't bring anything into this relationship. *So why not tell the truth?* I thought. I was a true believer in "Seek and you shall find." I had made no plans on making any unannounced visits to his new apartment trying to figure who he was dating. It was over. In the past, I had to learn the hard way.

As it got closer to Thanksgiving, I admitted myself back into the hospital as an outpatient for a platelet transfusion. This time they assigned me a room with another patient. They normally put me in a room alone because my immune system would be so low after chemotherapy. But since I was coming in for platelet and leaving afterward, there wouldn't be any harm.

I lay in the bed waiting for the nurse to give me two Benadryl capsules to relax me before the transfusion. The patient next me started coughing non-stop. I looked over at her, concerned if she was okay.

"Are you okay?" I asked.

"Yes, I'm fine," she said.

I thought. *Oh no! I hope I don't get sick. I just got finish with chemotherapy and my immune system is still very low. I want to be home during Thanksgiving holiday.*

I finally went to sleep, but when I woke up, my throat was so sore. The nurse came in to check my blood pressure and temperature. "Your temperature is up," she said.

"Oh really, but I'm feeling fine," I said. I was lying but I didn't want to spend the holiday in the hospital, I wanted to go home.

"Well, let me call Dr. Howard," she said. He might want to keep you in the hospital overnight.

No. I thought. "But I'm really feeling fine though," I said to the nurse. Unfortunately, Dr. Howard had to make the last decision if I could go home or not. The nurse came back, and she told me that the doctor instructed her to keep me until my fever went down.

A couple of days later, on Thanksgiving night, one of my friends, Horace, brought me a plate of his mother's Thanksgiving dinner. As he put my food on the tray, he gave me a hug.

"You're alone on Thanksgiving?" he asked.

"Yea, but I'll be okay," I said.

"Where's James?"

"Uh, he went to the Bayou Classic this weekend," I said.

"Oh," he said.

"I'm fine; we decided it best we went our separate ways," I said.

"DD, I didn't want to say anything, but he wasn't the man for you," he said.

"Now you tell me?" I said.

"I just didn't want to get in the middle of your relationship," he said. I wanted you to see for yourself.

"Oh, believe me, I have," I said. Horace sat and talked with me for a while, but I knew he had to be with his family also.

While I laid there on Thanksgiving Day, I thought how James was out enjoying his life while I'm fighting for mine. I always put others before myself. I always seat and listen to other people problems as I tried to help them resolve their personal problems rather than putting more faith in God and myself. I put a lot on my shoulders when I should've taken that energy and use it on myself so that I could've improved on what I wanted in my life.

One afternoon, when I was at home alone, I lay down because I wasn't feeling good that evening. I woke up feeling even worse. I could barely breathe. I went and sat down in the living room, thinking that it will eventually go away. It didn't help. I felt little light headed, and I still could barely breath.

I called the doctor's office that was on call that day. I spoke with one of his nurses. "Hi, this is Deagara," I said.

"Is everything okay?" she asked.

"No," I said.

"What's wrong?"

"I can't breath. Can I speak with my doctor because I think I need to be admitted back into the hospital?"

"Are you sure you want to come back in?" she asked.

"Why? I asked.

"Because I don't know how much of your insurance will cover," she said.

"What?" But I can't breath." I begin to cry.

"Let me call your doctor," she said.

She put me on hold for a couple of minutes. She came back to the phone. "Ms. Robinson, I just spoke with Dr. Howard, he wants you to admit yourself into the hospital," she said.

"Okay," I said.

And I'll inform the hospital that you'll be coming, okay," she said.

"Thank you," I said.

Once I got off the phone with her, I tried to contact James at work, but I only got his voice mail. I begin to panic because I was too scared to drive myself to the hospital. I simply sat on the sofa because I was still trying to catch my breath.

I sat on the edge the sofa and started crying again. "*Oh—God—what am I going to do?*" I asked myself. *God, please help me.* I prayed. I slowly pulled myself up off the sofa, I walked into my bedroom, and I put my tennis shoes on. I slowly walked out of my bedroom. I looked at the clock that stood on the dinning room wall. It was five o'clock in the evening, which meant rush hour traffic, especially on Frankford Road. I needed to get across to the other side of Frankford to go to the hospital. Frankford Road was one of the busiest streets during rush hour, and there was no traffic light around my apartments, so I couldn't wait at a traffic light. "*What can I do?*" I thought

I walked to my car thinking how I was going to get on the opposite side of Frankford Road. I got in the car and rolled all the windows down so that I could catch a good breeze of fresh air while I drove to the hospital. I held my head down toward the steering wheel as I prayed as I started my car up.

God, please let me get to the hospital. I'm so scared. As I backed out and pulled up at the stop sign, I looked down both sides of the street. Suddenly, I noticed that there was barely any traffic. I slowly drove across the street going west on Frankford toward Preston Road, and once I approach Preston the traffic light turned green.

I drove across Preston Road headed toward Coit Road, and I thought it was strange that each traffic light that I had approached the lights turned green at every intersection. Once I made a left turn on Coit Road, I crossed over the railroad track and proceeded over the Plano Parkway and Fifteenth Street intersection. And then I was there—the hospital parking lot.

I was relieved that I made it there. I walked into the admission area and took a set until one of the clerks behind the booth called my name. Once I was called, I walked over and sat down in front of her. She took one look at me, and she noticed that my face was very pale.

"Are you okay?" she asked.

"I can't breath." I said.

She got on the phone and asked someone to come down with a wheelchair. As I enter the fourth floor, they had a room assigned for me. I got out of the wheelchair, and lay down on the bed with all my clothes and shoes on. I was so weak and so relieved that I made it there safely.

A nurse came in a few minutes later, and she drew my blood for testing. As I was laid in a fertile position, the phone rang. I reached over and picked the phone up.

"Hello," I said.

"Ms. Robinson this is the Medical Center," a woman said.

"Yes."

"I'm calling to inform you that the National Registry has located two people that have the same protein as yours."

"Really," I said.

"Yes," she said. And we need to know if it's okay to check to see if their DNA matches yours?

"What?" I asked. I wanted her to repeat herself because I wanted to make sure I heard her correctly which she did.

"We've found two people on the National Registry that have the same protein as yours," she said. Do you want us to go ahead and test them?" she asked.

"Oh, yes please." I said.

"It's going to cost you a lot of money. It can be very expensive to get each one of these people tested."

I sat up on the edge of the bed. "But we're talking about my life right?" I asked her. She didn't say anything. "Can you please test them?" I asked.

"Yes," she said.

"Thank you," I said.

Later on that night one of the nurse walked into the room while I was still curled up in a knot with my back facing the door. "Deagara," she said.

"Yea," I said.

"How did you get here?" she asked.

"I drove myself here. Why?"

"Your test came back and you don't have any hemoglobin in your body."

"What? Oh really," I said. I didn't even know what hemoglobin meant, but they gave me a blood transfusion that night. I then felt much better.

The following night they gave me the okay to go home. The nurse that held my hand during my bone biopsy procedures was on the night shift that day. I told her the exciting new about how the National Registry found two donors who had the same proteins as mine, and they would be testing them to see if their DNA match mines.

She decided to walk down to the parking lot with me so that we could talk more. As we walked outside, it was raining, but we didn't care because we were both excited over my news. As we got closer to my car, we stopped and talked for a while.

"Deagara, this probably happen to you for a reason," she said. Maybe this had to happen to you so that you could probably help others understand this disease.

I thought, *maybe she was right because I did love people, and I was very compassionate toward others and what I believed in. Maybe I could make a difference. Maybe I could open some people's eyes or give others hope so that they could have a much clear understanding of Leukemia and how it affects people mentally, physically, and personally.*

On that rainy night, I took in what she said to me, and I started to think positive again. *Maybe God is giving me a second chance in life.* I was so excited by the news that I shared it with anyone who was willing to listen to me.

I still had to see my doctor on a regular basis. Nothing was final yet. I still wasn't in remission. The clinic had their own pharmacy in there facilities. I normally went there to pick up syringes that flush and clean the two tubes on my Catheter. As I stood there waiting for the pharmacist to bring back my items, I notice there was people sitting behind me. I heard them having a conversation about Leukemia. They felt that some doctors treated the disease as if it was a minority.

I stood there stuck because I wanted to hear everything they had to say. It was obvious they were concern for their lives or someone who was very dear to them. I looked back at them, and I realized they were four white couples. I smiled back at them, and I left. But I didn't forget their conversations or the concerns they had.

While I sat at home watching television, I was in a deep thought. I was still waiting to hear back from the medical center for the results. I still couldn't believe that they found someone in that short period of time. It had only been two months since I had been put on the registry.

I thought about how the doctor told me that there weren't enough African Americans on the National Registry and how he thought it would be a waste of time. While I waited, I decided to read the brochure again that was sent to me back in October about how the donor had to go through various tests before they could be donors.

James finally passed his real estate license. He was very excited. I began to notice that he came home a lot during the weekdays when he normally should have been at work. At first, I thought that he lost his job and didn't bother to tell me, but I felt that if there had been a problem he would've said something to me by now.

James walked into the apartment, and he didn't say a word to me. I notice he had walked into the dining room area and sat down at his computer desk. I heard him when he turned the computer on. I turned my head a little and watched him in the corner of my eye so that I could see what he was up to.

He put a CD in his hard drive. As he was prompting his feet on his desk, I turned back to watch television. He turned the volume up on the computer, and the volume got even louder to the point that it drowned out the sound from the television.

I didn't move, and I didn't even turn around. I sat there peacefully. He wanted to see my response, but I wasn't going to give it to him. The music got even louder. I could hear and even feel the vibration from the bass of his speakers that it got to the point that I couldn't hear the television at all.

I just sat there and I didn't move. I knew he wanted a confrontation, and I wasn't going to give him one. I sat there patiently until he realized that he couldn't get a rise out of me. He finally turned it down. I knew I was changing because normally I would've responded. However, now I had other things on my mind, and he wasn't one.

I called to check to see the status of the tests. She told me that once the donors past all required tests that she would notifying me. I was so nervous. I didn't know what to think. The test could come back not a match. The tested had come back from my siblings, and they were all negative. Mrs. Scott took Lauren in to a clinic to be tested. Hers came back negative, too.

So I had to seat and be patient and hope that things would go in my favor. While I waited, I ate everything in sight from being on Prednisone. My face was getting larger. I begin to have the symptoms of menopause for the first time. I would actually wake up drenched in sweat. I would take my temperature to make sure I wasn't running a fever again, which I wasn't. I knew then that it was a possibility that I was going into menopause.

One night I was in the kitchen washing dishes, it was around ten o'clock, and I heard James turning his keys in the lock. He walked through the front door, came to the kitchen, and sat down at the bar. I could tell he was upset. There was frustration written all over his face.

"Are you okay?" I asked

"I'm fine," he said.

"You don't look fine." What wrong?

"I just left a happy hour that my department had."

"Really," I said. Is this the same happy hour I ask you not to attend because you told me that they didn't like you?

"Yes," he said. They asked at the last minute and I told them I would.

"But something happen?" I asked.

"Yea, he said.

"What?"

"We were all sitting together having drinks and talking about work which it seems as if everyone was having a good time. Don't you remember me telling you about this young guy Tony that I didn't care that much for?" he asked me.

"Yea," I said.

"Well, he got pretty drunk."

"Oh really," I said.

"Well, when we all got up to pay the cashier for our tabs he walked up to me and said: "You know what, James? You ain't nothing but a wimp."

"What?" I asked "He flat out called you that?"

"Can you believe he said that to me?"

"What did you say or do?"

"I told him that I wasn't."

I hesitate for a second. "Huh?" I said.

"I told him flat out that I wasn't," he said.

"That's it? "I asked.

"Yea, he really made me angry! I stared at him as if to ask, *You couldn't have said more?* I stood in the kitchen waiting for him to say that he told this guy off, and he told him where to go but he didn't.

I shuck my head. We had a discussion early about him not going because majority of his department didn't care that much for him. "But, James, I told you not to go. You told me that they didn't like you." I said.

"DD, I got to get out of there," he said.

"James, we talked about this before, it's your move not mines. I told you a couple of months ago that you needed to fix your resume because you had too much information. But you told me that your resume was fine. Remember?" I said.

"Okay you're right," he said.

"Okay, then you needs to start making changes to your resume so that you can start sending it out to other companies," I said. Hopefully, someone will respond because it's obvious you need to leave that department or that company.

I knew he wanted me to do it but my mind was somewhere else. I wanted to find out my results, and I didn't have time for James anymore. I finally received a call from the nurse at the Medical Center; she told me that they found me a match from one of the donors with the same DNA. She went on to tell me that the donor had to agree to go through more tests. They wanted the donor to go through a full physical which is one of their requirements so that they can make sure the donor doesn't have any further physical problem that they weren't aware of.

She told me that she would be calling me back later for those results. I was so excited that I immediately called Mrs. Scott so that I could share the good news with her and Lauren. As I was talking with her, I heard the keys enter the lock of the front door. It was James; he had just made it home from work.

"Mrs. Scott, let me call you back." I hung the phone up and ran toward the front door. As he open the door, I stood at the foyer waiting to surprise him with the good news. "They found me a donor!" I said.

"Oh really," he said. I went to hug him as he barely patted me on the back.

He walked passed me headed toward the kitchen, but there was no reaction or excitement for me. With a nonchalant expression on his face, he said, "I knew they would."

"What?" I asked.

"I knew they were going to find you a donor," he said.

"How you knew?" I asked. I walked into the kitchen. I watched him open the refrigerator door, trying to find him something to eat. Eventually, he closed the door.

"How did you know, James?" I asked.

"Because you're a very strong woman, and I just felt that something good would eventually happen," he said.

"Huh?" Do you know how many people that are still looking for a donor?

"No," he said. He walked back to his room as I stood there shock because I didn't believe nothing he had just said because he never gave me any eye contact.

I thought about how I helped him with his real estate license when I was too weak and sick to hold my head up. But he couldn't give me any compassion about my well-being?

When he wasn't at home, I went into his room and found some hidden documents that he had up in his closet that showed that he sold his mother's house and that he received a large amount of money. Everything was beginning to make sense to me now. I knew how he affords a new computer, office furniture, and all those new clothes he bought home that day back in November for the Bayou

Classic. What I still couldn't understand was why his mother didn't have any place to live after he sold her house. Why was she living from place to place when James was sitting on the profit he made from her house?

I waited throughout the weeks to hear back from the nurse on my donor's results. During that time, I thought about when the nurses told me that the patient across the hallway from me had found his donor in Germany. I wondered where my donor was from. I knew I couldn't jump to the conclusions I just had to learn how to be patient and just wait until they call me back.

 I went in to visit with my new doctors that Dr Howard switched me to at the Blood and Marrow Center at Baylor Hospital in Dallas. I was nervous, but everything went well. The doctors were very nice. They ran a few tests and explained a little of the procedure about my bone marrow transplant. There were chances I could die from the procedure, which made me a little afraid, but I knew that with a lot of faith and determination I was going to do fine.

 That same day, I had a doctor appointment with Dr. Howard at three o'clock. I was so nervous because I had to get more blood drawn. They needed to check my white blood count to see if they were over a certain level. Once I arrived at the clinic, I went to the lab. Afterward I went to the waiting area, as I sat sending Christmas cards to some of my coworkers.

 As I sat there, I wanted to ask God, "Why Me?" But deep in my heart, I knew I still couldn't. It wasn't for me to ask. I was taught that God wouldn't give me something that he knew I couldn't handle. It wasn't for me to question him. But I thought this probably had to happen to so that it could make me even stronger in my faith in God and in myself. I just hoped that I could turn this situation into something more positive.

 The nurse called me to the back so that I could meet my doctor, but she had to first take my weight. This meant I had to get on the scale, which I've being avoiding for months. Once I got on the scale, I found out that my weight was up to 150 pounds from 135 pounds.

I followed the nurse to the back rooms and waited to see Dr. Howard. I sat in that room and I waited and waited for him, which made me so nervous because I didn't know what my blood result was going to say. A lot was going through my mind, as I tried to sit patiently for him to come through the door, but I was so afraid that he was going to bring me bad news.

As I sat there, I wondered, *What's next? What bad news will he be bring me, now?* When he finally arrived, he was very nice and cordial. "How was your visit with Dr. Sanchez?" he asked.

"It went very well, but they couldn't give me the actual date on when the bone marrow transplant would take place," I said.

I went into detail about my first visit at Blood and Marrow Transplant Unit at Baylor. Dr. Howard was very silent as usual. He stood and listened patiently to what I had to say.

"The reason why I'm asking when they're going to set up my bone marrow procedure is because I'm trying to find me an apartment before the fifteenth of January," I said.

"I couldn't tell you anything right now because I'm not for sure, he said.

Okay? I thought there he goes he's quiet again.

"So this will probably be the last time that I'll see you once Dr. Sanchez steps in as my oncologist? I asked.

"Yes," he said. They have their own oncologist at Baylor.

Okay he was quiet again. I thought to myself, *Okay, just shut up, DD.* I guessed I probably wouldn't see him again because I had questioned his profession during my frustration.

I told him that I was going to speak out about Leukemia. I wondered, *Did he really take me seriously?* I was hurt because he really had saved my life in his own quiet way, but I just didn't know

197

how to convince him or tell him how thankful I was that he saved my life.

It was a blessing from God that he was brought into my life. He was there for a reason, and I hoped that God would give me the opportunity to change the situation into something positive. Hopefully I would give others knowledge and hope as he had given me. I believed that God would show me the direction I needed to go, but I hoped he would show me how to express myself, as I talked about my trial and tribulations with others.

I received my bonus from my job. They turned around and gave me an extra bonus, which I thought was so wonderful of them. They always cared for their employees. We were spoiled. I admired the partners including the attorneys because they showed so much compassion and care for their clients and employees.

My coworker gave me a journal, and I put her card inside of the journal because it was so inspirational. It read:

DD–

How are you? We miss you! I hope you're feeling okay. Well, the wedding is about a week and half away. Boy—am I nervous. If you feeling up to it—I hope you can come! I bought this little journal for you several weeks ago. I thought you might need one during this time. It's always helps me to write things down. Also, you need to keep all this information and thoughts so when you write your book or become a speaker you have everything! God has a plan for you. Well, we are still continuously praying for you! I really miss you!

Everyday I began to write even more about what I was going through.

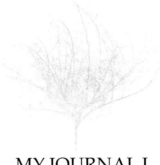

MY JOURNAL I

I thought, *If God is giving me a second chances in life maybe I can do my part as far as sharing what I felt throughout my struggle with Leukemia.* I decided then to make the best of the journal my friend gave me. I started writing everyday what I was feeling and what had occurred.

December 30, 1997

It was getting closer to the end of the year, which was very slow for me. I made plans to do a lot of cleaning, but as usual, I found myself not getting much done. I guess this day was not that day. I was so tired that I lay down for a while until I received a called from Joseph, Lauren's father.

He wanted to inform me that his lawyer needs hundred and eighth-nine dollars from him to start the processing fee so that his wages could be garnish for child support. When he told me all this information over the phone, I thought finally we could discuss this matter without going at each other's throats. I didn't say as much. I just listened.

I didn't want to be confrontational with him anymore. I felt that I had to put closure to this matter because I was more concern about my life. It's seems that all that fussing we did in the past wasn't worth it. I guess something like this had to happen to me so that I'm able to move on. I also realized that I had to make peace with myself first so that I can move on with my own life.

I thought, at first, it would be very selfish of me to think about myself first and not others. But, I knew I look at it differently. God has always blessed me in so many ways, even without the financial or moral support I needed from Joseph. God was always there for my child and me and that's where I'm going to keep my faith.

I really didn't receive much from Joseph when it came to child support, which was fine with me. I realize now where all my blessing were coming from, but I knew I needed to learn how rely on God and not on flesh anymore. They would sometimes disappoint you.

As the conversation went on that night, Joseph started to discuss his trip home in Florida during the Christmas holidays. I sat on the phone, and I didn't say a word. I just listened to what he had to say. That was something I was still learning to do. Maybe, if I did more of that, I probably could have gotten a better understanding of Joseph and his family.

As I listened to him discuss his trip home, I knew what he was going to discuss next.

"I took Lauren Christmas shopping while I was in Florida," he said.

"Oh you did that was nice," I said.

"She did so well in school. I asked her what she wanted, and she asked me was it okay if she could get a second set of holes in her ears," he said.

"Oh really, okay," I said.

So where is your man?" he asked

"I don't know," I said. I guess he's at work. But let me stop you right now because we're not going to discuss him. The phone got very quite.

"You know you can get great airfare if you go through this company," he said.

"Oh really," I said.

DETERMINATION

I realized as I sat on the phone that I was changing because I didn't fall into his trap. I was in control.

The next day, James came home from work pretty early, around one o'clock that afternoon. I thought it was strange because he never came home for lunch. As he walked through the front door, I noticed he was wearing casual clothes rather than his work clothes. I knew he was having problems at work, but I began to wonder. *Did he lose his job?*

He was very quiet, and I didn't go out my way to speak to him. I had already fixed myself something to eat so I got up, took my plate into my room, and closed the door. After I finished eating, I walked back into the kitchen and I noticed he tried to bake a potpie. As he pulled the potpie out of the oven, I saw the crust was burnt.

I put my plate in the sink and walked back in my room. Within fifteen minutes, he was out the door and gone. Around two thirty that afternoon, James decided to call me.

"Hello," I said.

"Hey, has the electric bill come in yet?" he asked.

"No." Not yet. I said. But I should receive the bill around the fifteenth of January.

"Oh okay," he said. The phone went silent.

"James, if you're so concerned about the electric bill you can pay sixty-five dollars for utilities, and whatever the difference that is left over, I'll pay it myself," I said. At that point, I decided if he was in such a hurry to leave then I was going to give him a quick exit.

I didn't need him because he was never there for me while I've been sick. Even though I loved him, I could go on without him and not even be angry or have any resentment toward him.

I felt that only God was going to pull me through this difficult time. I knew that things might look bad for me right now, but I knew that he always came in at the right time to smooth things out in my life.

Even though it's very hectic for me right now, I was very frustrated that I hadn't heard from Baylor University Medical Center about the exact date of the procedure. The last time I spoke with them, they told me that they'll let me know something a week in advance with a definite date. I just hope it's after 15th of January so that it'll give me enough time to move into my new apartment.

My mother told me that she'll come back down to take care of me during the procedure but she couldn't give me a definite date though, but she wrote me again:

Dear Dee,
I hope you had a nice Christmas. I was unable to call you.
I don't feel welcome using other people phones sometime. Your brother told me that I need to get a phone in my house, which I will soon. I love you and I pray for you. Whenever you want me to come, I will be there for you. I wish I could go through this for you. You're strong with God by your side. I'll be there as long as you need me. I love you so much. I'll call.

After I read her letter, I decided to call her at my grandfather's house. My aunt had brought my mother a house that was a couple houses down the street. My grandfather had someone walk down to her house to get her for me, as I waited on the phone. Once she came to the phone, I told her that I got her letter, and that I was sorry she had to use other people phones, but I told her that I needed her because I was afraid after the hospital explained the procedures. She told me that she'd be there when I needed her.

I called Southwest Airline and used my VISA card to set-up a date and time for my mother's airline ticket. I instructed the airlines to have my mother's tickets waiting for her at the airport in case she decided to come at a later time. They explained to me that they have to charge me a late fee for the delay, which I was fine with because I just didn't want to see my mother riding the bus again and having to beg a total stranger for a ride to my home.

DETERMINATION

December 31, 1997

It was nine thirty in the morning, and there was a knock at my bedroom door. "

"Hey, DD," he said. It was James.

"Yea," I said.

"Hey, I've put half of the rent on the kitchen counter."

"Oh okay." It was obvious he was in a rush to move out. This would be the last time he had to pay to live in this apartment. As I laid there in bed, I thought about how I once wrote out a check to him for the rent and the same day the check was cleared through my bank.

How would he feel if I went directly to his bank like he did me? Would he think that I didn't trust him, too? But that wasn't me. *I'll let his check run it course through my bank.* I now understood that there was never any trust in our relationship.

Not once did I go to him for money. I knew me and I knew the faith that I had in God. If James ever needed me, I would actually be there for him, but I had to ask myself, *Would he have done the same for me?* In the back of my mind, I already knew the answer.

I don't think James knew how selfish he really was. When it came to his own personal things or his own emotions toward others, he really didn't know how to share them. He held on to all of his personal belonging, and he treasured them without being able or willing to share unconditionally and I don't think he knew how.

I was the opposite. Even though I didn't have as much, I knew how to give unconditionally. I didn't expect anything in return because it made me feel so good inside and I knew deep inside that I was always blessed by God. He had always provided for me and my child so I knew I was blessed

Later on that day, I ran errands. I went to my bank, the clinic, and to the grocery store. On my way home, I went by the leasing office to pay the rent, and I stopped by the post office to pick up our mail. Once I got back into my car, I put the key in the ignition. It wouldn't start.

"No! What's going on?" I sat in the car for a while. Then I tried to start it again, but it did nothing. I walked to the apartment I notice there was a message on the answer machine. I listen to the message it was James. I hit the button.

"Hey, it me," he said. "I'm just checking to see if you found my check on the kitchen counter?" As I listen to his messages the phone rung. I picked the phone up.

"Hello," I said.

"Hey," he said.

"Hey."

"Did you get my check?" he asked.

"Yea I did," I said.

"Is everything okay?"

At this time, I put my pride to the side. "My car won't start," I said.

"Is it your battery?" he asked.

"I don't know. It's not turning and it not making a sound at all."

"Well, I get off at six o'clock tonight. I can look at it then when I get home but are you speaking to me?" he asked.

"Why?" I asked.

"You haven't said anything to me all this week."

"What do you mean?" I asked.

"I thought you weren't speaking to me," he said.

"No I'm not angry with you. It's just that I have trust issues with you, that all." The phone went silent.

"Well, I'll be home soon," he said.

"Okay," I said. We hung up the phone.

It was seven in the evening. I sat in the living room wondering, *should I go ahead and calls a mechanic so that they could tow my car to their shop? They'll probably charge me fifty dollars for the towing fee. I guess I'll wait until James gets home.* I knew I needed transportation to get back and forth to the hospital before he moved out and when we went our separate ways because after living with him for six months I knew I couldn't rely on him.

It's seven-thirty p.m.; he hadn't made it in from work yet. W*here is he?* I thought. *It shouldn't take him this long to get home from work; he's only fifteen minutes away.* There was a knock on the door. I looked through the peephole. It was James. I open the door, and he walked into the apartment without saying hello to me.

He was very quiet as he walked passed me headed toward his room. *"Okay?"* I thought. *Is he not going to ask me about my car?* As he was walking into his room, I followed him into the hallway and I stopped.

"James, are you still going to look at my car?" I asked.

"Let me get undress," he said.

We walked around the corner to the mailbox where my car had stopped. His car was already parked by my car. He popped his trunk open where I noticed he had already stopped by Chief Automotive for a new battery, two jumper cables, and a flashlight.

As we walked toward my car, he went on the driver side and sat down. He tried to start the car, but it still wouldn't start. He popped open the hood, walked up to the front of the car, and open the hood. "DD, you need to learn how to change your battery in your car," he said. I didn't say anything.

"Plus, you owe me money for the battery and the jumper cables, too," he said. I still didn't say anything. I just stood there as he messed around with the old battery. I thought how he tried to impress me when we first started dating me. He took my car in to get it detailed one day, and he surprised me by new car mats for my car. Back in the real world, I thought, *Hey, if he's willing to help me with my car, I cannot complain. I'll pay him.*

We stayed outside for almost an hour, as I held the flashlight and he tried to get the battery out of the car. The cap that connects the battery was stuck, and he was having a very difficult time getting it off. I started feeling guilty for the way I was treating him by not saying anything to him for almost a week. He could've stopped working on my car, but he was determined to get the cap off.

I finally knew that he really cared about me, even though we were going our separate ways. I figured we would probably be there for each other as friends. We'd said some things out of angry. I wish I could've taken some of the things back, but the damage was done. Just like, James we are both trying to find ourselves, but I guess this had to happen for both of us to realize that we weren't meant for each other.

He finally got the old battery out of my car, and he put the new battery in within a second, as the car started. I was so excited and relieved because I thought it was probably something major wrong with my car.

"How much do I owed you?" I asked.

"Nothing just for the parts," he said. We walked back to the apartment, and I went to the kitchen to start dinner because that Prednisone was doing it job on me. I was so hungry.

James walked into the kitchen and gave me the receipt for the battery and jumper cables. "Here the amount you owe me for the parts," he said.

"Oh okay," I said. Thank you. I didn't say another word after he hand me the receipt because I rather pay for the parts than a mechanic for parts and service.

As I was cooking dinner, James walked back into the kitchen. "DD, we need to talk," he said. I turned around.

"Why?" I asked. I'm cooking us dinner.

"I'm moving out this weekend or the following week," he said.

"Oh okay, that's fine."

"DD, we tried but it didn't work out."

"I know."

"I found a great apartment on the third floor that's away from everybody," he said. It was very quiet and very peaceful area, and there's a lots of trees behind my apartment. Plus, I'm not paying above my means either. It's nice apartment with a den.

"Well, good for you," I said. I'm happy you were able to find something that you could afford.

"I don't want us to leave being angry with each other," he said.

"I understand," I said. I really do, and I'm happy for you. I'll always have love for you, James, but we should be just friends. I know that now.

I turned back around to the stove and started back cooking. I wanted James to understand that by me being stricken with Leukemia that the relationship we had was a learning experience for me. God had taught me to appreciate life more even though I'm moving on to better things in life. I felt that he really didn't understand that I'd already moved on when it came to him.

I was sitting at the bar eating my dinner when James came back into the kitchen. "Have you found a place yet?" he asked.

"Yes." I said. He waited to see if I would go into any details, but I didn't. I could tell he wanted to know more.

"So how much are you paying for your rent?" he asked.

"Six hundred and five dollars," I said.

He shook his head. "That sounds like something you would do," he said.

"You get what you paid for," I said.

James never brought up the name and location where his new apartment located, and I was not going to ask for it either. I hadn't told him that his new manager called the apartment by mistake so I knew exactly where he was moving to but I didn't care.

"So can I come over sometime for dinner?" he asked.

"What?" I asked.

"Are you going to invite me over to your new apartment for dinner?" he asked. I didn't say anything. I just shook my head.

I thought, *Could you believe this man? Does he actually think he* could come over to my apartment at his convenience when he wasn't willing to let me know where he lived? "I don't know right now," I said.

Later on that night, I took a good look at myself in the mirror. My face was big and round like a large pie. My belly poked out even further. I stood there hoping that one day that things would change, and it would go back to normal again. But I had to be honest with myself and realize that my life was never going to be the same again.

January 1, 1998

Well, it a New Year day. It's twelve o'clock in the morning. I received a phone call from Horace. "Happy New Year, boo," he said.

"Happy New Year to you, too," I said. Where you head, tonight to a party?

"No." I'm headed to church."

"Oh…really, how nice. Maybe next year I'll be able to go to church too."

"You will."

"Well, you be careful out there."

"I will. Are you okay?" he asked.

"I'm fine," I said.

"Well, I'm just checking on you."

"That's sweet of you." We hung up.

In the middle of the night, James came in my room, which I thought was strange because he normally stuck his head through the door when he wanted something. "Hey, will you do me a big favor since I fixed your car?" he asked.

"What?" I asked.

"Will you help me with my resume?"

"Sure, when?" I asked.

"I'll let you know," he said.

"Just let me know when you're ready, James," I said. We can do it together.

I woke up early on New Year's Day once the phone rung. It was Lauren calling me to wish me a Happy New Year. I was so happy to hear her voice. She called to let me know that she loved me, but as usual, we just held the phone not saying as much.

I've noticed when my daughter called me we don't have as much to say to each other after I ask her how was school or was she having fun down in Florida. After I asked her those questions, we didn't say much. We went quiet as we held the phone. We were becoming strangers. I loved her so much, and I miss her so much. I prayed that God give me a second chance to raise Lauren because I knew she was going to need me more as she got older.

She gave the phone to Mrs. Scott, we talked for a while, and we hung up. After I got off the phone, I went to the kitchen to start breakfast. I had a taste for pancakes, bacon, and sausages for breakfast because as usual my appetite was out of control.

As I started cooking breakfast, James came into the kitchen. "You have a minute?" he asked.

"Yea, sure what wrong?" I asked.

"I need to talk with you," he said.

"Okay." He sat down at the bar.

"DD, I'm concerned about my job. I'm so unhappy because the management in my department is very bad. I can't stand my new supervisor. He has been in that position for only a month, and he had the nerves to call me into his office to express to me how he thought that I wasn't a team player in his department."

"Oh really. Why?" I asked.

"I really don't know, DD." He barely speaks to me. So when he walked pass my desk. I don't say anything to him," he said.

"But James this has been going on for several months now. If I were you, I would've looked for a new job a long time ago when he called you in their office pertaining to your performance. That was a true sign that you should've been looking for a new job," I said.

"I need set hours because I'm tired of working on the weekends."

"James, we went over this before you need to fix your resume."

"I need something better than what I have right now."

"Yes, I have to agree with you but you should've done this a long time ago." I stood there in the kitchen, as I listen to him complained about his job. He tried to convince me the troubled situation he was in. Then he got up from the bar.

"I need to make some phone calls," he said. Let me get started on that right now.

"Okay," I said.

"Will you help me with my resume?" he asked.

"Sure, James," I said. He got up from the bar and went back to his room. I sat down, and I ate every pancake, two slices of bacon and sausage patties that I could put on my plate. After eating all that food, I decided to clean up my mess. James came back into the kitchen about ten minutes later.

"Hey, DD," he said. I turned around from cleaning the stove.

"Yea," I said.

"It's official," he said. I just got off the phone with the apartment complex. I'm moving out on the January 4

"Oh…okay," I said. *What is he up to?* I thought. I just couldn't put my fingers on it. The apartment complex should be closed on New Years Day. I didn't trust him. I figured out that he was all about himself. In time, he'd show himself.

As I was cleaning the kitchen, James came out of his room with his Play-station controller in one hand and his keys and pouch in the other. "I'll see you later on tonight," he said.

"Okay," I said. He walked toward the front door, but it was obvious that his resume wasn't that important *If things were so bad*

DETERMINATION

at his job, he should've at least get his resume out of the way before he moved in three more days. I would've thought.

An hour passed when James knock on the front door. I looked through the peephole and wondered why he was so lazy that he couldn't use his own key to open the front door. I guess his friend wasn't at home. I opened the door, and I let him in.

"I'm so tired," he said as he walked into the apartment.

"I almost fell asleep at the wheel; I need to get some sleep," he said. He went back into his room and he closed the door.

I put some clothes on and ran some errands, but it wasn't much I could do because mostly everything was closed. I went to the grocery store to purchase black-eye peas and pork chop for dinner.

When I returned home, James was still asleep, but because he was a light sleeper, I guess he heard when I came home. Approximately thirty minutes later he walked pass my bedroom with the same items in his hands. "I'll see you later," he said. I thought, *What about your resume? Oh well, I guess I'll spend another special day alone.*

Later on that night, I cooked black eye peas, fried boneless chicken, and baked some cornbread. It was delicious, too—all three pieces of the fried chicken. But I forgot to take my Prednisone before eating my meal. At the time, my stomach was full. I couldn't eat anything else, but I knew I had to take my Prednisone with either food or milk.

I decided to drink milk with the medication. I drank the first glass of milk, and it was good. So I decide to drink a second glass of milk, which it really did a number on my stomach. I was so sick that I had to lie down. I went in my room, and I curled up in a knot. I was in so much pain.

I couldn't even sit down or stand up. It got so bad that eventually I couldn't even lie down. I sat on the edge of the bed, as I tried to read an interesting book that I bought from the grocery store. It was a book on women's health, and it talked about how stress played a major factor on health and how important it was to have social and moral support from family and friends, which I didn't have.

As I read this book, it got me to thinking that I was really alone. I realized that I didn't have any family here with me in Dallas that I could call on for moral support. Instead, I had chosen to isolate myself away from others because I didn't want my problem of being sick to be their problem too.

I didn't want them to feel that they were obligated to be there for me because I didn't know if I was going to live or die. After reading that book, I realized that I needed to learn how to live a stress free life and learn to make friends, who were supportive of me and me to them.

After drinking two glasses of milk my stomach was really hurting me. "Okay, okay," I kept repeating. I tried to lie down again for a while, but before I could lie my head down on the pillow, the doorbell rung. I knew it was James. This time he didn't knock; this time he decided to ring the doorbell.

As I slowly went to the door, I looked up at the clock. It was almost two o'clock in the morning. I was in a lot of pain as I walked toward the door. I opened the door to let him in. I proceeded back to my room to lie down. He followed me into my room and lay right down beside me.

We lay facing each other in bed. He began to talk to me. "Can we talk?" he asked. I took a deep breath "Sure," I said. Even though I was in a lot of pain, I was curious about if he was going to bring up the discussion about his resume again. I just lay there and listened.

"I'm concern about my job. I hate my job so much because I don't understand why I'm having such a difficult time there. Plus there are not enough blacks at this particular branch, especially at the Plano location. I think they were being prejudice toward me because I felt like they enjoyed picking on me a lot," he said.

As I lay there listening to him, I remembered when we had first met. He had told me how his last job was prejudice toward him too.

They can't be prejudice at both places, I thought. *I think he needs to take a good look at himself.* I interrupted him.

"James, let me stop you for a second," I said. You can't blame the city or the people for what's going on in your life. I think it's the people you're probably coming in contact with and it might be something you're doing wrong too. If this consistently happens to you then maybe it's you? I asked.

As he tried to explain his problems, I wasn't going hear anymore of it. "James, it's just that you haven't come into contact with the right people!" Don't you be so quick to make judgments because you've had bad experiences on your job because things will turn out better for you but you have to make those changes in your life too? I said.

"Anyway, if it's that bad at this company, the first thing you need to do is clean up your resume up. You have too much stuff on your resume. Plus, most employment agencies like to look at a one-page resume. That way it's very easy and quick for them to read. I have been telling you this for months, and you wouldn't listen to me. As you put it, "*My resume was fine. Don't touch it.*" Remember? So now it's a rush, huh?" I asked.

I was getting mad, so I got up. I sat on the edge of the bed, but I was still in a lot of pain. I looked back at James with disgusted on my face. "James, I told you to let me look over your resume six months ago, and I was willing to retype it for you." I said.

"We can do it tonight," he said.

"I'm not feeling good tonight, maybe tomorrow," I said.

He wouldn't stop talking. I lay back down on my back. I eventually turned my back toward him with both of my hands clutching my stomach. Not once did he ask me what was wrong. I tried my best to tune him out but as I lay there. I thought, *If I didn't drink that second glass of milk I wouldn't be in so much pain.*

I crawled up in a knot, and he still didn't ask me what was wrong. I just couldn't believe he wouldn't stop talking. "At my old job, when

I use to work at this insurance company, my supervisor had a big crush on me. But I didn't go that way," he said.

"What you're talking about?" I asked. Why you didn't go that way?

"What?" he asked.

"Was she was white?" I asked.

"Yea," he said.

"Oh boy—please," I said.

"But she had a crush on me, but I didn't respond to her. So she tried to get me fired. She made my life difficult while I was there."

I said to myself, *Enough*

"I'm sick!" I screamed. I'm really sick! He looked at me with shock on his face. He got up and immediately and left the room. As usual, I had to sit on the bathroom floor for a while as I got on my knees and waited until I finally threw up.

January 2, 1998

I woke up early that morning screaming. I had a cramp in my leg. "Oh God!" I screamed. It hurts so badly! James rushed into my room. "Are you okay?" he asked.

"I have a Charlie horse," I cried. He went into the bathroom, and he got a warm towel and placed it on my right leg. I thought that was nice of him to make an effort after I had scream at him earlier.

My conscious began to mess with me. I felt that I should help him with his resume, even though I knew he was playing games. I knew that he only wanted his resume done before he left so that he could put distance between us.

Back when I was trying to get over Raymond, Mrs. Richards was my inspiration. She had given me so much wisdom just by me being around her and listening to her talk about taking my hands off situations that I really didn't have any control over. She was the

DETERMINATION

one who told me, "You can't do right in God's eyes, so don't expect him to answers."

I could hear her now: "Dee, take your hands off it, baby. God always has a way of fixing the problem. It might not happen when you want it to, but he'll fix it where you can see it." That's how I got my revenge when someone did something to me. I'd kill them with kindness because I knew I had something even stronger watching over me.

I realized that I couldn't pass anything by God because he had a way of working things out at the right time. I wasn't worry about getting revenge at James. I was just going to take my hands off it and try to do right by him because God was going to make the last judgments because it wasn't for me to do.

That morning, I got up and fix me a big breakfast with grits, eggs, two slices of bacon, and flaky biscuits. While I was cooking breakfast, James came into the kitchen. "Can we talk?" He asked. I begin to roll my eyes, thinking, *Okay, here we go again*. I didn't even turn around. "Yea sure," I said.

He sat at the bar while I cooked. "I decided I was going to try to get transferred to a different department at my job, but I need a resume to send in with my request form," he said.

"Okay," I said.

"But my supervisor has to sign off on this form to give me the okay to transfer."

"Well why you can't provide them with your current resume you already have now?" I asked sarcastically.

"No, I rather have an updated resume," he said. I thought to myself, *Here…we go again! He's playing games. Why is it that he just won't come out and ask me to help him with his resume? Oh—No! He wants to play games.* I was tired of this.

A couple of months ago, he didn't want to listen to me when it came to his resume when he wasn't getting any responses from other companies. I thought, *I just got finish preaching to myself about* *putting this in God's hands, but he's really making it difficult for me to keep my faith. I am not going to let him get the best of m*e.

As I stood there in the kitchen cooking, I started praying to myself. *God forgive me if I'm wrong, but I don't want to be anybodies fool anymore. He said he was there for me the time when I was at home running a fever and I couldn't breathe, I had to drive myself to the hospital. He wasn't there. I don't know how to handle this God? I don't.*

January 3, 1998

The next days I turned the ringer off on the phone so that I could get some sleep. When I finally got up I noticed on the caller id, there two calls from James. I didn't return his phone calls. However, later on that evening when he called again, I picked the phone up.

"Hey!" he said.

"Hey," I said as I took a deep breath and sighed.

"I'm just calling to see if your battery was working okay in your car?" he asked.

"Huh?" I said. Yes its working fine. But I'm thinking about taking it in for an oil change and tune up on Monday. Why are you asking?"

"I just wanted to make sure everything was fine with your car," he said. *Hmm*—I knew what he really wanted to know, but I wasn't going to bring it up.

James came home around 7:30 that evening. He came into the apartment in a very joyful mood. "I'm going running, and when I get back, we can start on my resume," he said.

"I'm sorry James, but I'm working on my book. I'll let you know when I have the time," I said.

He came back from running, and I noticed that he was pacing through the apartment most of the day. He washed all of his clothes. He was slamming the doors and cabinets. He turned the television up very loud. He finally came in the kitchen where I was writing. He went into the refrigerator to make a sandwich. "I'm going in here and go to asleep for a while. Will you wake me up?" he asked.

"Sure," I said. But I was thinking, *May he sleep in peace.*

The phone rung; it was Horace calling me from his car phone. "Hey, boo," he said.

"Hey what are you up to for tonight?" I asked.

"I'm headed to the movies to see *Amistad.*"

"Oh that's nice. Are you taking a friend?"

"No, I'm going alone."

"Oh okay."

The phone was silent for a second. I walked to my room and shut the door. I kept the lights turned off as I sat on the floor against the wall. "Are you okay?" he asked. At this time, I broke down in tears.

"Horace, you know when someone is trying to be manipulative and sneaky about things rather than being up front with you?" I asked.

"Yea," he said.

"Well, I'm so tired of feeling guilty because of this crazy relationship that I'm in right now. I'm sick and I'm sitting here waiting for a call from the hospital about my bone marrow transplant procedure that I'm going to have soon. I have to go through more chemotherapy. I've been poked on so much that I'm just tired. I'm tired of the games that I have to deal with when I come home from the hospital. Horace, I'm sick and it seems like he doesn't care." I said.

"Boo, it's going to be okay. Just do what you have to do," he said.

"I'm sorry for crying," I said. I hope you enjoy the movie. We talked for a while and we hung up.

Once I walked out of my bedroom, James was standing in the hallway. "Are you okay?" he asked.

"Why?" I asked. He knew that I just got off the phone with Horace. He probably heard every word that was said, but I didn't care if he heard me or not. I was too angry to care.

I looked him straight in the face and I didn't even blink an eye. "I'm tired of the game, James," I said. You're being sneaky.

"What are you talking about?" he asked.

"You have been going on and on about your job and how you're so unhappy. Now you want to hurry me up on your resume before you move out. You must think I'm stupid?" I asked him.

"You are always assuming things, DD. That's not my intention," he said.

"Look!" I got a lot on my mind. If you haven't noticed, I'm sick! I'm about to have bone marrow transplant, but I don't know when. I could actually die from this procedure, but at the same time, I have to move soon into my own place. So I don't need you to play these dumb and manipulative games with me, James," I said.

"DD, you're not going to die," he said. But I don't like you to be on the phone discussing anything about me. They're going to judge me before they have a chance to meet me," he said.

"Your sneaky, James!" I said. You won't be up front with me and that's what hurting me.

At this time, it was one o'clock in the morning. We both calmed down and began to talk to each other more civilly. It seemed as if James was being very understanding and caring. "I really need your help with my resume," he said.

"Well, come on, James." I said. Turn on your computer and let's get started.

As he turned the computer on, I went into my room and I pulled out my resume books. He brought his desk chair from out of his room so that I can sit at his desk. When I was using his computer to start on my book, the chair suspiciously appeared in his room.

But as I sat down to begin on his resume, I could tell he was getting frustrated. "I'm so tired," he said. Would it be okay for me to take a nap for thirty minutes and I promise I'll help you?

"No!" I said.

"Only thirty minutes, please?"

"You can lie on the sofa because I'm going to have some questions that need to be answered by you," I said. I could tell he was unhappy, but once he lay down he fell asleep, as I typed through the night.

By five o'clock in the morning, I was almost finished with his resume. I created a one-page resume so that it was easier for the viewer to glance at key words and his major skills. I fixed the fonts, bonded the heading, and set the margins, but the only thing I needed from James was his objectives. "James, wake up!" I said. He pulled his head up. "I'm almost finished with your resume all I need is your advice on your objectives," I said.

"DD, I'm so tired," he said. I got to go to work in the morning. He got off the sofa, and he walked back to his room and closed the door.

I thought, *You fool! You fell for it!* I went to bed feeling hurt that he used me. I eventually calmed myself down, and I went back and finished his resume by putting his old objective onto his new resume. I was hurt to the point that I wanted revenge. While I sat at his desk, I tried to put his resume on my disk and delete it from the hard drive, but I couldn't find one. So I saved it under a new name where he couldn't locate it.

MY JOURNAL II

January 4, 1998

It was six in the morning, and I couldn't sleep because of the Prednisone. I use that time to write my book. I was really mad. I was so angry that I was talking aloud. "Let him search for it!" I said.

But my conscious messed with me. "No." Let him know where his resume is." My conscious kept saying, *"Vengeance is mines said the Lord."* I printed out a copy of his resume and placed it on the kitchen counter where he could see it when he got up in the morning. I went back on the computer, and I saved his resume on his hard drive so that he was able to locate it.

It was now eight thirty, I heard James walking out of his bedroom. I rushed to my bedroom door. As he walked passed my door, he came back into the hallway and stopped. "Hey, did you see your resume?" I asked.

"No, I haven't. I haven't had a chance yet," he said. He walked to the kitchen and glanced at the resume for a minute. "This is nice," he said. He gave me a pat on the back.

"I appreciate this," he said.

"You welcome," I said.

Around ten thirty James called. "Hey, I'm hungry can you bring me something to eat?" he asked.

"What do you want?" I asked.

"Could you stop by Subway and buy me a sandwich with chips?" he asked.

"Okay but I need to first stop by the bank to get some money," I said.

He never asked me to bring him food to his job before and he never invited to his office before. *So why now?* I thought. But I thought since I told him I would I'll do it. I really didn't want his coworkers looking at me in a strange way because of my pie face. Was he setting me up so that one of his coworkers saw me? I didn't know what to think. Maybe I was being a little paranoid, but again I didn't trust him.

As I got in my car to start it, my car hesitated for a second like it didn't want to start. "Not again." I thought. *It's probably my alternator. I have a new battery.* I took my car down the street to Goodyear. I sat there for a good hour an a half before they were able to look at my car. They couldn't find anything wrong. In a way I was glad my car acted up because I didn't want to feel embarrassed when I took him his food. It cost me some money for the mechanic to check my car out, but I didn't fall into one of James little games.

After I left the mechanic, I ran a couple of errands while I was out. I went to the grocery store and to look at another apartment complex because I haven't heard from the other complex. I decided to go to Pear Ridge Apartments off Frankford Road. The manager took me to look at some of their apartments. I thought they were very nice. The person that was in the leasing office was very nice too.

I explained my situation to the manager that I was about go through a bone marrow transplant procedure in a couple of weeks, and I needed to know something soon so that I could move before that time. She was very understanding and asked that I filled out

DETERMINATION

an application and to put down a deposit fee, and she'd tell me something soon.

I filled out the application and left a deposit. After I left there, I tried to think of somewhere I could go so that I wouldn't be there when James moved out today but it didn't work out that way. As I drove up and got out of my car, James was backing a U-Haul into the parking lot. I got out of my car and walked into the apartment. I thought, *It is actually official; he is moving out today.* I was hurt and little angry because I was going to be by myself, even though I knew it was over.

I took the cordless phone in the kitchen in my room, and I closed the door. I could hear him and his friend moving his bed and boxes out of the apartment. It didn't take them long to move his furniture and belonging because he never really contribute anything toward the apartment, mostly everything that was in the apartment was mines.

After he finished moving his things, he came to my bedroom door and knocked on the door. I open the door. "Hey, I'm gone," he said.

"Okay," I said.

"I want you to know that I've learned a lot from you."

"And I've learned a lot from you too, and I wish you the best, James. I really do." I said.

After he left, I walked into the master bedroom; it was totally empty. I could hear an echo as I opened the closet door to see if he left anything behind. He was really gone. I shared this room with him for a couple of months. I didn't cry though I was hurting inside. I mostly felt loneliness, but I knew deep inside that this was for the best. I needed a peace of mind so that I could try to get myself together.

Later on that night, I got a lot done. I clean up the apartment. I even organize my personal papers, and I, finally, I got some rest. I thought, *Well maybe I'll start missing him down the road, but right now, I don't.* I was enjoying being by myself. I was able to think things out in clearer perspective rather than worrying about a man who really cared about only himself.

For once, I slept for a long time without any interruptions, and it felt good.

January 5, 1998

It was three o'clock in the morning, and I couldn't sleep. I guess the Prednisone was keeping me up again. I was having hot flashes, too. Since I couldn't sleep, I got up and cleaned the hold house up. By five o'clock, I still couldn't sleep. I finally decided to lay down again when I realized that I was really tired. I woke up around eleven. I felt much rested.

I called the hospital myself since I hadn't heard from them. I spoke with Lisa, doctor's assistant, who I thought was very caring person, and she provided me all the information that I asked for or what needed to know.

Lisa told me that she thought the donor was a man, and she explained to me that they asked him to go back to the clinic again for another full physical exam before he could donate his bone marrow to me. I was a little upset. He had gone through this before. *Why should he do this again?* But she explained to me that the donor was very understanding that he was willing to go in today for more tests.

I was still upset and worried because the donor had already volunteered to go through various tests with the other hospital. "I'm sorry, Lisa, but I was just wondering why they have to keep putting him through this?" I asked. He already went through the procedures before."

"That's part of the procedure," she said. We want to make sure everything was accurate since your doctor switch hospital to Baylor.

"Oh," I said.

"Plus, we have to make sure that his DNA actually matched

yours," she said. We think that your Bone Marrow Transplant will probably take place within two weeks.

Really, I thought. *This would give me enough time to move into my new apartment, and I could get myself situated too.*

After I got off the phone with Lisa, I sat thinking that whoever this donor was. *He must have a good heart and he has to have very good patient to go through this again for me.* It seemed that he has a lot of love and faith in God to be doing this for me. I felt so blessed.

January 15, 1998.

Finally, the day had come. I was officially moving into my new apartment. I had been waiting on this for a while. I was ready to get situated so that I didn't have to worry about it while I was in the hospital. As I was moving my things, the hospital called me that they wanted me to come in the next day for some tests so that the insurance company can approve the bone marrow transplant.

"Tomorrow," I said.

"Yes," she said. Your doctor also wants you to come in to do a bone marrow biopsy. *Not another bone marrow biopsy.* I thought.

"Will I get something that will put me to sleep because I've been pocked back there at least four times?" I asked.

"If you request it we will be happy to give you something."

"Yes, please."

"Could you be in at one thirty tomorrow?" she asked.

"I'll be there," I said.

The move went smoothly, and the apartment was beautiful. The apartment had plenty of light. By me still taking Prednisone on a daily basis, I had so much energy that night I was able to organized my entire apartment. Even though I had to be at the hospital the next day, I didn't sleep at all.

January 16, 1998

Once I got at the hospital, I waited for thirty minutes before the lab technician called me into their lab. As I walked in, they asked me to take a set in one of the chair that stood against the wall. The chairs looked like a school desk. I gave her my right arm to draw my blood, but this time I didn't turned my head around. I sat and watched her as she filled my blood into these tubes. I wasn't afraid anymore. I was facing my own personal fears.

While I was sat there, she explained to me that they needed a urine sample from me within twenty-four hour. They provided me a plastic cup that was sealed in plastic bag. "I need you to pour your urine into this container and keep it under ice in the freezer," she said.

Can I put it in an ice box?" I asked.

"Sure you can do that also," she said. I thought *I don't want my own urine in my refrigerator where I place all my frozen food.*

She instructed me to go back in the waiting room until I was called to the back to see my doctor. Within another thirty minutes, one of the nurses called me to the back. I followed her through the door. "Hi," she said.

"Hi," I said.

"How you're doing today?" she asked.

"I'm fine."

"Before I can take you back to see your doctor, I first need to take your weight," she said.

"Oh okay. Can I take off my shoes?"

"Sure."

I stepped on the scale and stood up straight so that she could get an accurate count of my weight. I was curious to see how much I weighted. I looked up toward the ceiling as she messed around with scale. "You weight 159 pounds," she said. I looked at her with shock on my face. *What happen to the 135 pounds five months ago?* I thought. I guess it was gone for good.

I followed the nurse into this small room and sat down on the examining table as she took my temperature and blood pressure. She put a line in my arm for the biopsy procedure because I asked my doctor at Medical Center of Plano to remove the Hickman from my chest for a while. I just wanted to feel like myself for a little while until it was time for my bone marrow procedure.

About fifteen minutes later, I followed her into another room where she asked me to lay down on this table that stood against the wall. "I need you to turn your back toward the wall," she said. But as I got on the table and I turned my back toward the wall I realized that there was a window there not a wall which was a good thing because I could look out the window and look out toward the sky wishing that I didn't have to go through this again.

I was so afraid that the Leukemia was back. I got so paranoid because whenever my current doctor would do the biopsy the results comes back that I wasn't in remission. I lay there looking out of the window crying. One of the doctor's nurses came into the room to introduce herself to me, and she noticed that I was crying.

"Are you okay?" she asked.

"Yes, I'm fine." I said. I tried to wipe away the tears from my eyes, but I couldn't stop crying.

"I'm sorry," I said. It's just that I've had bad experiences in the past that all. She patted me on my back to try to comfort me but it got to the point that the tears wouldn't stopped falling. "I'll be right here, okay," she said.

Eventually she left the room for a minute. As I lay there, I begin to pray to God to give me strength to overcome this fear that I was having and to think of a positive outcome. The doctor's nurse came back into the room.

"Ms. Robinson, we are going to try to fix it were you don't have to take the bone marrow biopsy," she said. We are going to try to use the December biopsy for insurance purposes. Okay?"

The tears fell from my face with relief. "Okay. Thank you," I said.

After a while, my doctor came into the room. He explained that he would rather do the biopsy right now rather than later because he would have to do it anyway once I was admitted into the hospital. "I just want to go ahead and get that out of the way so we don't have to worry about it later, okay?" he asked.

"Okay," I said.

"I will be right back okay," he said. Thank you.

The nurse stayed behind. "Will someone be able to drive you home after the procedure?" she asked.

"No," I said. I drove myself here.

"I don't think we can give you this drug to relax you doing your procedure," she said. Let me speak with the doctor.

The nurse came back in the room. "The doctor explained to me that he's going to wait until later because the drug is too strong for you to try to drive yourself back home," she said. I thought the doctor was very understanding, but I suddenly felt that I needed my mother. It made me realized how important family and friends were.

By the time I walked down to the garage to get into my car, I was in tears. I was so angry with my mother—and myself—because she wouldn't give me a definite date on when she was coming. In the back of my mind, I knew she was coming because she loved me, but I needed her so much right now.

When I got home, I left a message at my brother's house to let my mother know I needed to talk with her and it was very important that she called me back. By this time, I needed someone to talk to because I was hurting, but I didn't really have someone personally to call on. Horace was so busy with his job, and I didn't want to bother him.

I decided to call Mrs. Scott. I felt she was very understanding and helpful during this time of my life. While we were talking, she explained to me that my mother loved me and I needed to give her a couple days. We sat on the phone and talked for a while. "Dee, if I would've known you needed someone I would've of came down myself," she said.

I thought that was very nice of her to be willing to do that for me, but I felt that she was doing enough for me by watching my baby for me. After I got off the phone with Mrs. Scott, I felt much better. I knew that God was always there for me, and I hoped that in the future that I can confine in him more and to learn to be patience enough to wait until God knows what's best for me.

January 19, 1998

It was seven in the morning, and I finally finished with my twenty-four-hour urine test. I can take it back to the lab at the hospital. I had an eight thirty appointment to meet with the medical imaging department, where they were going to run tests to see if my heart was strong enough to go through the bone marrow transplant procedure.

I drove to the hospital, and I sat and waited for about forty minutes with other patients who were waiting patiently to see their doctors, too. Eventually, the nurse called me back into the hallway, where there was a bed against the wall.

"I need you to take off your jacket and lay on the table there," she said.

I hesitated at first because we was in the hallway where there were people passing by. I felt somewhat weird laying on a bed right out in public, but I didn't say anything. I just did what she asked.

I got up on the bed, and I lay there for a good fifteen minutes before she came back with two tubes in her hands. "I'm going to take some of your blood, and then inject this medication into your arm for testing. After thirty minutes, I will inject your blood back into your arm therefore we confirmed how strong your heart is," she said.

She rubbed my arm with alcohol and stuck the needle in my arm. It was so painful that I turned my head toward the wall as she drew my blood into the small tubes. After she drew my blood, she injected this medication through my arm which I could feel the fluid from the needle enter my veins.

"I need you to wait in the waiting room until we call you back," she said.

"Okay," I said. She left the needle in my arm so that she could inject my blood back into my arm.

Within thirty minutes, she called me back to a room where I sat down under a machine. She re-injected my blood back into my arm. "Now we can test the muscles in your heart to see if everything is okay," she said. I'll be right back, okay.

"Okay, thanks," I said.

As I lay there for a while, I felled asleep. She came back into the room. "Ms. Robinson," she said.

"Yes," I said.

"You okay?" she asked.

"Yes. I'm sorry, I guess I'm tired," I said.

"That's fine, she said. Please wait here. I'm going to let the doctor review the results okay. I thought, *She seems to be a nice person. I should've jumped to conclusions so fast because I thought she was too straight forward in the hallway earlier.* Within fifteen minutes, she came back into the room.

"You can go now," she said.

"That's it?" I asked.

"Yes."

"How did my test look to the doctor?"

"Everything looks great."

"Okay, thanks."

My next visit was with my social worker. I had an hour an a half to waste, so I ate lunch in the hospital cafeteria. I tried to find a place where I could hide from others because I was ashamed of my appearance. After I had my lunch, I walked over to this building to meet my social worker.

Once I entered the building, I walked downstairs to a basement. As I entered the hallway, there was a library and a conference room on the left sided of the hall. I was unsure if this was in the right

DETERMINATION

place that I needed to be. At first, I thought I was lost. I walked further down the hallway, and I noticed three women working in this large room.

"Excuse me," I said. Hi. They turned around.

"Yes?" One of them said.

"I'm sorry but I think I have a meeting in this area," I said. I was told by my social worker would be somewhere down here.

"You're in the right location," One of the ladies said. Let me page your social worker because I think he's probably busy with another patient.

"Okay. Thank you," I said.

When I finally met my social worker, he was very nice. He asked me if it was okay if one of his students from Romania can set in to listen to our discussion. I said I was fine with it. "So how are things going?" he asked.

"Everything is fine with me," I said. But I feel that I need moral support. I sometime feel that I needed someone to listen to me and I didn't have that. I start crying.

"I'm sorry for crying but I know sometime I talk too much," I said.

"It's okay. Please don't apologize. I'm glad that you're saying what you're feeling. I can get a better understanding on how we can help you that way," he said.

He begins to ask me questions that I couldn't really answer. "So what do you do for fun?" he asked.

"Well, I like to spend a lot of my time with my daughter, and I love to shop." I said. But I then said to myself, *You know what, DD? You don't put anytime for yourself. If I'm not working, I'm running arrange, getting Lauren settled down and situated after spending the summer with her grandparents, or getting her ready for school for the next day. But I don't know how to have fun, but I need to start.*

After I spoke with my social worker, I had to go back down to my car in the garage to get the cooler that had my urine specimen in. Once I arrived in the bone marrow center, I gave the urine test to the lab. I sat their in the waiting room for my appointment with the doctor, and later, I learned that I would be meeting with his assistance.

She explained that the doctor will be using a different type of chemotherapy during the procedure, and if I would come back after the orientation tomorrow, she would tell me what type of chemotherapy the doctor will be using then which I told her that will be fine.

I left the hospital headed for my next appointment with my current doctor in Plano. I was in such a good mood. I felt that everything was looking up for me. I finally expressed myself to my social worker for the first time, which was something I usually kept to myself.

Once I arrived to the clinic in Plano, I had to go to the lab so that they could draw my blood for more testing. I went back into the lab. As the nurse was drawing my blood, she accidentally dropped the tube. She rushed to get paper towels as she kneeled down to wipe the blood off the floor. "I apologize," she said. I'm so sorry.

"That's okay," I said. I was in such a good mood that it didn't bother me that she dropped my blood right in front of me, even though it meant that she had to draw more blood.

I had to go back in the waiting area. While I waited, I decided to write some letters to some of my friends. Once they called my name, I followed the nurse down the hallway so that she could take my weight. I was now up three more pounds. "You looked so unfamiliar since you gained so much weight," she said.

"I feel like the Pillsbury dough girl." I said. She started laughing.

For the first time, my doctor arrived early into the room. I explained to him what went on today. "Good," he said. Let me check your blood in the lab and I'll be right back.

Once he came back into the room, he said, "It looks like two of your cells look funny. They look like damage cells from so much chemotherapy, but they didn't look like Leukemia cells," he said.

The good mood was gone. I got scared again. And my doctor knew it. "I'm sorry you looked as if you were in a good mood," he said.

"That's okay. I would want to know the truth. If it were Leukemia, would you have told me?" I asked. He shook his head to reply to say yes.

"If it would come back now, it wouldn't matter because you're about to have a bone marrow transplant which it's going to wipe out all your own bone marrow and you will be receiving someone else," he said.

You stated to me that I have a fifty percent chance of the Leukemia coming back. Is it still that percentage? He couldn't give me a clear answer. I decided then to leave the percentage thing alone, but as I walked out of the clinic, I was disappointed and hurt. I started talking to God because I knew only he can pull me out of this. *"God, I know this is only the devil." But I know that you are with me but it hurts because I don't know when to be happy or sad.*

When I made it home, I decided to call Mrs. Scott because I knew she would know what damage cells were. She said there were such things as damage cells. As we talked, I felt better, but even though it was still in the back of my mind, I knew it wasn't much I could do but to rest my mind.

January 20, 1998:

I had to attend an orientation at the hospital where they showed us slides on what to expect during my bone marrow procedures. She told me that my donor wasn't a he but a she.

"Really," I said.

"Yes," she said. And she very excited about giving you her marrow.

"Really—," I said. I begin to cry. *That was nice. She must be a wonderful person.* I thought.

She gave me and another patient a tour of the floor where I would be located during the bone marrow procedure. She explained that our doctor like for us to move around to get exercise or participate in some type of craftwork they would provide us during our stay. Most of time I was there my mind was somewhere else. I was so frustrated that I hadn't heard from my mother.

When I arrived home, I called Mrs. Scott again because I needed to talk with someone. I didn't know what was going on with my mother. I didn't know if she was coming or not. "Be patient with your mother." Mrs. Scott said. "Your mother is coming; I don't think she'll let you down. If she doesn't come then I'll come and stay with you until you get better or until you can handle it on your own."

"No, Mrs. Scott, I'll be fine." I said.

"Dee, you're going to need someone down there with you," she said. I was still hesitated but I wasn't given up on my mother. We might have our differences, but I knew she'd be there for me eventually.

I spoke with Mrs. Scott for a while, she asked me to let her know if my mother haven't came at a certain time or a particular day and she will be there for me. When I got off the phone with Mrs. Scott, I decided to call my mother and she was at home. "Momma, when are you coming to Texas? I begin to cry.

I was so scared that she would have to delay. "Tuesday," she said.

"Oh…okay," I said. I felt good knowing that she put a date on when she'll be here. We talked for an hour. I was happy and relieved to hear from here especially when she would be able to arrive in Dallas.

As I said my good-byes to my mother I wrote down her new phone number, James beeped in. "Momma, I don't want to hold you on the phone too long plus James is on the other line. Let me see what he wants." I said.

"Okay," she said. I'll call you tomorrow.

"Okay. I love you momma."

"I love you too," she said. I beeped over.

"Hey," I said.

"Hey, what are you doing?" he asked.

"I just got off the phone with my mom." Why?

"I was just wondering if you could take me grocery shopping later on today."

"Huh?" I said.

"I need to learn how to eat health, DD," he said.

"Oh. Sure," I said. But I thought *James only calls me when he wants something from me. I guess he's trying to get whatever he can out of me so that he doesn't have to ask or see me again. I could just feel it, but time will tell.*

When he came over, we lay on my bed reminiscing about the past. We laughed and joked for a while. I asked him was there any way he could help me assemble my treadmill I purchase once I had my bone marrow transplant, but he kept bringing up grocery shopping. We finally got up and left. We stayed in the grocery store for about two hours.

I went to the airport at Love Field waiting at the terminal until everyone got off the plane. I stood there watching anxiously, and I finally saw my mother walking out of the terminal. We smiled as I gave her a hug. I was so happy to see her. Once we got back to the apartment, she got situated. She decided to sleep on the sofa because I only had one bed in the apartment. I felt bad, but she wanted me to be comfortable.

February 2, 1998

I had a one thirty appointment with the radiation doctor. I was instructed that someone suppose to be personally escorted me over to the Radiation department. It didn't happen that way. I went to the bone marrow area. They did more lab work on me. I remembered that the date was getting closer for my bone marrow transplant. I was beginning to get scared because I knew I could die from the procedure.

When I arrived at the Radiation area, the nurse was standing, waiting at the front door for our arrival. I followed her to one of the room so that I could meet with the doctor. "I need you to take off your clothes but just the upper part of your body, like your shirt and bra," she said. The doctor needs to check the upper part of your body.

"Okay," I said. I did as instructed.

Once the doctor arrived, he explained some of the side effect that might occur from the radiation. Such as my chances of having another child would be slim because the radiation treatment would leave me infertile and a high possibility I would have early menopause.

"Menopause? I thought you get menopause in your fifties," I said.

"Yes, after six months you won't have a period," he said. They'll probably give you hormone pills to control some of the symptoms from the menopause. There's a good chances of you developing cataract which corrective surgery may be recommended later on.

'There's also a twenty percent chance of another type of cancer reoccurring down the road," he said. *What!* I thought, *You get rid of one cancer and another might occur?* I didn't say anything. I'd wait and discuss it with my oncologist later.

He also explained to me that I would lose my hair within two weeks of the treatment. He said that my hair would not return until three to four months because of the radiation, but because of the low dosage, I might be receiving my hair back sooner.

The doctor left the room for approximately fifty minutes when he returned with his nurse. They checked my eyes and body for any swelling. After the doctor checked me over, another nurse came in and measured me from head to toe and took a picture of me so that they could keep up on how the radiation would have an effect on me.

When I left the radiation department, I went back to the bone marrow center where the head nurse was waiting for me. I followed her in one of the rooms so that I could visit with my doctor. As she was checking my blood pressure and temperature, I asked could my mother join me in the room, which she thought would be okay.

My doctor came in, sat down, and asked me if I had time to read over some documents and contract they had provided me. I stated to him that I've read the contract three or four times. "Do you have any questions?" he asked.

"Yes, I have one question," I said. Do I have a chance of developing another type of cancer later on in the future?

"It really applies to patients who had breast cancer, lymph, etc, which it would sometimes come back ten years later with another type of cancer due to the radiation," he said. But he explained with Leukemia it was a slim chance because of the lower level that I would be receiving, but they had to tell me the percentages.

Once I got home and we got settled, I decided to call Mrs. Scott. She was becoming an inspiration to me. She was always positive and very motivating when we talked. "How's Lauren doing? I asked.

"Oh, she's doing fine," she said.

"How's she doing in school?" I asked.

"She's working hard, and she's trying real hard too." I could tell in Mrs. Scott's voice that Lauren was still having problems in some of her classes.

"She does well on her lessons, but when it comes to tests, she does okay," she said. "Oh…okay." I said.

"Have she been to the dentist yet since she been down there with you?" I asked. If not, I could give you her insurance card.

"Actually, she has a dentist appointment next week," she said.

"Do you need her insurance information from her card?"

"Oh, we've already have insurance for Lauren."

"Oh really, that's good," I said. So does Joseph have insurance for Lauren?

"No, Carl and I have insurance for Lauren," she said.

"Oh, okay then." I said. Good.

"So when do Lauren get out of school?" I asked.

"Sometime in June," she said."

"The reason I'm asking is because once the bone marrow procedure is done and I'm back on my feet, I need to spend some quality time with her before she goes back to school."

"I could understand that you need that time with her," she said. The conversation became very short when we started discussing Lauren. I knew then I needed to get my child back with me as soon as I could.

I knew it was going to be very hard to unattached Mrs. Scott from Lauren, but I knew that my child needed a lot of discipline and guidance in her life. She was about to be a teenager, and she was going to need me badly. I also knew that I had to teach my daughter how to put God first in her life, which was what I was learning now.

"Can I speak with Lauren?" I asked Mrs. Scott.

"Sure," she said. Lauren! Your mom wants to speak with you. Lauren came to the phone.

"Hello," she said.

"Hi, Lauren," I said.

"Hi."

"How's school? I asked.

"Okay," she said.

"So have you made a lot of friends while you been in Florida?"

"Yes."

"Have the little boys been trying to talk to you?"

"No," she said. Well one guy.

The phone went quiet. We didn't have that much to say. I was somewhat hurt because when she was in Dallas with me, we would talk about everything. This time our conversation was very short. Tears started rolling down my face. My baby would not open up to me. I held in my emotions so that she wouldn't think anything was wrong. "GG's here," I said.

"She is?" she asked. You can hear in here voice that her spirit lift up when I said my mother's name.

"Yea, do you want to talk to her?" I asked.

"Yea," she said. I gave the phone to my mom. They spoke for a while then my mother talked with Mrs. Scott. I really didn't want my mother to speak with her because I didn't want my mother to start saying anything negative toward me or come off in a negative way.

I sat on the side of the bed crying. I was so hurt my daughter wouldn't open up to me. I began to realize how everyone else had control over me—and my daughter. Everyone was happy except me. I always felt that when I was diagnosed with Leukemia that God did things for a reason. I never question him as to why this happened to me but I was beginning to realize that I had to make me happy, and I needed to take control of my own life because I only had one life to live.

After my mother got off the phone, I went back into the living room so she could comfort me. "Momma my own child wouldn't even open up to me," I said.

"That's just how Lauren is," she said.

"But we usually can talk about anything, we were so close," I said. My mother was quiet for a while.

"Mrs. Scott said she was going to bring her down to Dallas so that I can see here," she said. *What!* I thought.

"I don't want my daughter to see her mother suffer," I said. She's not bringing Lauren down here right now. Not during my bone marrow transplant procedure, Momma. Lauren is coming home in June, and if I have to call Mrs. Scott, I will.

As I got up off the sofa and walk toward the bedroom. "Next time don't you call me!" she screamed.

I was hurt and mad. I went into the closet and fell to the floor. I start crying aloud, where she could hear me. I wanted my mom to come in and comfort me. To hold me and ask me what was really wrong with me. Or just come in and hold me tight and tell me that everything was going to be okay but she never came in.

As I lay on the floor, my conscience began to talk to me. *"DD, you are looking in the wrong place." "God will always be there."* I realized that only God was going to see me through this. That I need to look for my comfort through God and not through another person which he has created. I can't put all my trust into another person because there's a chance he or she will let you down. Only God would always be there when I needed him. He always came right in time.

"I will take control of my life God." I thought. *I will start praying to you God so that you can help me bring a lot my closure to you and I'll learn to put you first in my life and not your creation, because they are not perfect and neither am I but God I need closure. I have lot pain that I'm dealing with but I'm going to let you fight my battles for me God.*

I got off the floor. I decided that I had to put off writing my book but I kept writing in my journal. I felt that God has blessed me in so many ways; he had always been there for me. He had always come right on time when I thought there was no way I was going to get through some of my problems throughout my life.

I really didn't have any one to talk to personally because every person had their problems too, but God, always has time. All I had to do was to get on my knees and pray and talk to him. My friend Horace told me that God had a way to bring me closer to him, and slowly but surely, he was doing that now.

February 3, 1998

Today, I had to meet with a surgeon who was going to place

DETERMINATION

a new Hickman back in my chest. I already had three different procedures regarding where to put the tubes on my chest. It had left several scars, which I hoped to clear up with coco butter.

Once we left the hospital and we return home, my mother wanted to go shopping, window-shopping as she put it. I gave her the keys to my car and I let her go on her merry way. I had more concerns than shopping.

While my mother was gone, I called Mrs. Scott to ask about my daughter coming to Dallas while I was sick. "I told your mother that once you are home from the hospital, I'll bring her to Dallas to see you," she said.

"No, not while I'm sick, Mrs. Scott," I said. "I don't want her to see me this way. I want to be up and about before she comes home. I'll see her in June."

"I understand your decisions, DD," she said.

We talked for a while and then we hung up. Mrs. Scott was such a positive person. She had a way of taking a negative situation and switching everything into something positive. These past months I felt very close to her because she listen and understand what I was going through. She let me cry, and she gave me her opinion without saying anything negative toward the other person. Before I got off the phone with her, I let her know that I appreciated that she listened to me and that I felt very close to her.

February 4, 1998:

I was awake from a call from James. I was half sleep when he called. "Hey, you're sleep?" he asked.

"Yea," I said.

"Do you want me to call you later?" I know you're going in tomorrow but I'll call you later.

"Okay." I said.

Once he called me, I was up. All I could think about was running errands and making sure that my mother had funds until she received her income tax. The phone started ringing constantly.

My coworkers were calling wishing and praying that I make a quick recovery from my bone marrow transplant.

The hospital called giving me directions to admissions. They set up my appointment for me to be there at six o'clock in the morning. The surgery will take place at seven thirty, and they instructed me not to eat anything for twenty-four hours before the surgery.

I received a call from James again. By this time, everything was piling up—the calls, getting my finances situation before I went into the hospital. Plus, I had to pack my pajamas and other items that I needed while I was in the hospital. When I heard his voice, I was in tears. I wanted to pour out to him, but I knew he wouldn't listen to me. But I held everything in. We talked for only a short time because I was so choked up.

"I need to go by our old apartment complex to return my keys," he said. I felt that he wanted to ask to come by, but because I was so short with him, he didn't know how to ask. "Well, I'll talk to you later," he said.

"Okay." I said. I felt guilty; I immediately called him back and asked could he come by? He said. "Yes."

Within thirty minutes, there was a knock on my door. It was James. "Hi," he said. He came in sat down on the sofa.

"How are you?" he asked.

"Fine," I said, but I really wasn't.

He sat glowing, looking at the television and not once at me. "I've been working out and I was able to transfer into a new department at the company and my new job is going great," he said.

"Good." I said. As he talked to me, he would never look my way. *I know I have gain a lot of weight, but am I that ugly to him now? I* thought. *It was a time where he couldn't keep his hand off me.*

He finally asked me what was wrong. I told him how irresponsible my mother was being because she took Clorox to clean a spot off the rug. "Well you need to sit down and have a long talk with your

DETERMINATION

mother," he said. But once he said that I could tell by his expression that it wasn't his problem.

I was getting angry because he was being selfishness and self-centered. So I got up and sat at the bar. He got up from the sofa and walked over to my treadmill. "So, I see you got your treadmill assembled," he said. Now, he has the nerves to get on it after I asked him to help me. Now, I was really pissed. He got off the treadmill and came and sat by me as he made a statement. "We always had a communication problem," he said.

"*What!*" I thought. *We could talk about events, politics, joke about each other, our goals in life and you say we have a communication problem. He really knew how to say the wrong thing. He can say something so low down to you and stay calm with it that really got into your skin.*

"I don't want you," I said. Believe me I don't. I looked at him for the very first time and he looked so ugly to me with his high top, half-parted hair-do that he had just got done by his barber.

As he sat at my bar with those polyester pants on, he wanted to say we have a communication problem. "James I want you to know that whenever you need me, I hope I'll be around because I'll be there for you even though you wasn't there for me emotionally or mentally," I said. I won't do you the same way you did me. I promise you that.

"I got to go!" he said. I don't want to hear none of this.

As I watched him walked toward the door, I became so angry because he really didn't care about me. I got up from my chair and ran toward him with my hands balled up in a fist. I hit him in his back. As he turned, I grabbed for his face. His glasses fell off. He grabbed me, and he threw me on the sofa.

I got up and went at him again as he ran toward the door. "You're crazy!" He screamed.

"I'm not crazy!" I screamed. I'm just angry how you treated me! I never hit a man or a person, but you made me so angry. I'm sick and you don't even care! Just then, I hit him again. He grabbed me again and shoved me toward the wall. I summoned all my strength and hit him again. He finally grabbed the doorknob and rushed out the front door.

I was so terrified. *Why did I let that happen?* I asked myself. *Why did I let him get the best of me? You fool! Why?!* That was only the devil in me. I immediately call Mrs. Scott. Her phone was busy. Within fifteen minutes, Mrs. Scott called me.

"Are you okay?" she asked.

"No." I said. I just jumped on James. She began to laugh.

"Mrs. Scott he made me so mad. I never fought or hit a man, but he came into my apartment with an attitude that he didn't care even though I helped him through his personal problems.

"Dee, James has to go through something because it's obvious he doesn't understand what you're about to go through." She began to laugh again.

"You know people write books about you," she said. *"A Woman beat up on Their Man."*

"No, Mrs. Scott it seems that he was gloating as if he had his life ahead of him." I said. And what I'm going through is not his problem and he didn't want to understand. If he cared or loved me like he said he did then he would've listened or tried to give me his personal opinion and confidence that things were going to be okay, but he can ask that of me though.

"I thought if we were truly friends we would be there for one another even if he was dating someone else we should still be there for each other because of the past experience we had. I thought that we could at least been friends. But oh no—he wants to cut ties where he didn't want to deal with my disease." I said.

I thought about James' mother who had divorced his father years ago. Whenever she saw him they would gets into a fight. *Why?* Had he hurt her so badly with his manipulative ways? Is this a genetic problem with the men in this family? Why would his mother carry so much anger unless he had really hurt her in the past? *Maybe God is saving me from future pain.* I thought.

As Mrs. Scott and I were talking, my mother walked in the front door. She had just made it back from the hair stylist. Her hair was beautiful. "Mrs. Scott, my mother just walked in the door," I said. Can I call you back later once I'm in the hospital?

"Sure," she said. Good luck.

"Thanks." We hung up.

I told my mother about the incident that had occurred between James and me. She didn't say anything at first. "Why did you do that?" she asked.

"Momma, he made me so mad," I said. I felt that he was gloating about his life when I was about to go in for my bone marrow transplant. She was quiet. She didn't say anything for a while.

I began to cry. I felt that my mother would rather support someone else than her own child. As I sat at the bar, I realized she would never change. She would never support me when I really need her to. I thought she knew that James treated me badly, but with the negative comments she made of him in the past, it wouldn't have made any different if James was treating me well.

Later on that night, while she was cooking ground beef on the stove, she turned around and looked at me. "You know what?" she asked. Whatever you did for James, you can't expect anything back in return if you were sincere.

"Momma, James and I went through a lot together and I thought we were supposed to help each other so that we could get ahead," I said. I felt that I was used. No, Momma. Because if he was in the same predicament I'm in now, I would've stood by him. I began to cry but I knew I wasn't going to win this argument so I left the conversation alone.

I had several errands to run before I admitted myself in the hospital, I decided that I wanted to send out Valentine cards to my friends and family. My mother and I stopped at *Lord and Taylor* to shop before we arrived back to the apartment.

Once we made it back home, I received a call from the anesthesiologist, who had to ask me several questions before the surgery tomorrow. "I don't like to wake up during the surgery because I'm known to wake up when the doctors haven't finished the procedures," I said.

"So you want to sleep throughout the procedure?" he asked.

"Please," I said. I begin to cry.

"I really appreciated it." I said.

"Try to get some sleep early, Ms. Robinson, and don't eat anything after twelve o'clock," he said. Okay, I'll see you in the morning.

That night I decided to budget my checkbook and forward money from my savings to my checking to cover the checks I wrote at Lord and Taylor. I went to the grocery store, and I wrote a check for cash so that my mother could get tokens for the garage at the hospital. I went to get gas and saw my dream car—Mazda Millennium. I wanted to remember something positive before I went into the hospital before my procedure. If I made it through the bone marrow procedure, it was my goal to buy a Mazda Millennium for Christmas. That was going to be my own Christmas present for myself.

When I returned home, I finished packing. I couldn't sleep, so I stayed up until it was time for me to go to the hospital. While I was up waiting until morning, I watched a Christian channel on cable. There was as couple whose wife was diagnosed with cancer and relapsed twice, but she did not give up. She had so much faith in God that she knew he would always be there for her.

However, what really touch me was one of my favorite NFL athlete was on the show too. He went into details on how God changed his life, and it was an inspirational feeling for me to realize that God always has a way to bring you closer to him.

February 5, 2006:
Since I was up, I washed my face, put up my clothes on, and woke my mother up. I notice it was raining outside. I went downstairs to put my luggage in the car while my mother was dressing. When we arrived at the Surgery Center, I sat with a representative who asked me various questions.

Once they called me to the back, I changed into a surgical gown and slipped on the house shoes that looked like socks. I had to take out my contacts and earrings. The nurse showed me to this waiting room where my mother was waiting for me. I asked the nurse if they would automatically admit me into the hospital. She stated she was unsure. I became very frustrated because I had to go back into surgery again and I didn't know what was next.

It was time for my surgery. They walked me in this room, where I had to lie on a table as they wrap my arms around some sheets. They put monitors on various parts of my body to watch my heartbeat. The anesthesiologist stood over my head. He noticed that I was teary eyed. I began to feel a stinging feeling in my hands.

"I'm feeling a burning in my arm," I said.

"That's the anesthetic," he said. Within two seconds, I was out.

I slept through the surgery. When I woke up, I was in the recovery room. I wanted sleep but they forced me to wait up. I noticed the Hickman was back in my chest. This time there were three tubes rather than two and they were very large.

Eventually I was strolled to the fourth floor where the bone marrow transplant would take place. I slept most of the day, when I woke up, I tried to turn I had a lot of pain in my right arm I had to request for anesthetic from the nurse but once the anesthetic wore off, I was still in pain.

When the phone rung, it was hard for me to reach for it I was in so much pain, I just let it rung. The bed, which my mother was supposed to sleep on, was like a recliner chair. It was no way my mother was going to sleep in that chair. "Momma you sure you don't want to go home?" I asked.

"No, this will be all right." she said. But after a while, she thought about it again and decided to go home and come back in the morning.

My doctor explained the procedure to me, which I had to go through almost three days of chemotherapy and two days of radiation. By this time they swiped all my blood cells they would give me my unrelated donor's marrow that will make new blood cells. They also explained that my body would try to fight off the new cells because they were foreign to my body, which I would be under doctor's care for a year.

The day I supposed to received my donor's marrow, I was so scared and very nervous. Anything could happen when the courier tried to transport the donor's marrow. A nurse and the courier brought the cooler into the room. I didn't know what to expect.

As they open up the container, I noticed what I thought to be was blood. They put the bag of marrow on the pole and they connected the IV to my catheter.

"That's it?" I asked.

"Yes," she said. What did you expect?

"I don't know," I said. I guess I thought that when you talk about bone marrow they had to remove a bone or something.

"No," she said. They took her bone marrow from her lower back where your marrow produces also.

"So basically, it as like a blood transfusion?" I asked. She smiled, and she said yes.

The courier told me that the donor's family was so thrilled to help me. She hand me a gift bag, which had a stuffed animal inside, two letters one for me and another for my mother, and an inspiration book, *Chicken Soup for the Surviving Soul.* Inside she wrote:
With our wishes for you and your family, God Bless from your donor and her three children. February 12, 1998.

I noticed there was a handkerchief in the bag, and there was a note tapped on the handkerchief that read:

My mother always told me to have a white linen handkerchief in my pocket—here is one for you with Love!

I open the envelope, and I read her letters to my mother.

Hello,
    I have thought of you and your family daily since I first learned that we have this special project together. Though you're suffering, you have given me such a gift, and I want thank you for that. When I learned that my three year old daughter had Leukemia, I felt that if I lived to be 150, I could never repay all the kindness that was shown to my daughter. Somehow before I left the hospital the first time, I became determined to focus on every good thing that happened.
    The sicker she was from the chemo, the more convinced I became that the medicine was working. There have been few things I have looked forward to more than this. When my child was so sick, I never actually prayed for her life. Somehow, I knew her life was in God's hands. I did pray hard and deeply for the quality of her life, for her strength, and for guidance. How was I ever going to explain hair loss to a three year old? Together we did it! She has always faced life with courage and determination. Life itself is a gift we can all share. Looking at my gorgeous child instills such hope and pleasure in me. I am so very fortunate.
    My mother is also a cancer survivor. It is for my daughter and my mother that you and I now have a bond. Life throws us many changes; somehow, we must look deep within ourselves and find positive little things in life to keep us focus.
    God Bless, 2/12/1998

Within a couple of weeks, I was released, and my mother was with me throughout my treatment. I was so weak. I didn't have any energy, and I didn't have a taste in my month. My mother tried to get me to eat, but I just didn't have an appetite. Every morning she had my medication laid out on this tray that was next to my bed. She drove me to the hospital every other day, which was so tiresome, but she drove without complaining.

Once we got to the center, I had to go to the lab as I sat and watched them draw my blood, as my mother waited in the waiting room doing her needlepoint. Whenever I had to have a blood or platelet transfusion, she and one of the nurses, who was on lunch break, would sit and talk until it was time for me to go home.

I was getting so tired of going to the hospital. My feet and ankles were so swollen that I could barely walk. By the time we walked up the hill in the garage and got into the garage elevator, I was exhausted.

"I'm tired, Momma." I started to cry.

"I just want to die," I said. She started crying because she knew I was suffering.

"Don't talk that way, Dee," she said. She hugged me. It's going to be all right.

One night, I noticed that my skin was pealing. "Momma, something is wrong!" She ran into the bedroom.

"What's wrong?" she asked.

"My skin it's pealing," I said. Why is it doing that?

"I don't know," she said.

The next day we went to the Center my mother, and I showed my doctor my skin on my legs and certain parts of my body. He told us that it was Graft vs. Host Disease. Because my donor was from an unrelated donor, my body tried to fight off my new marrow. He told me that my color should come back within months.

A couple months passed, and I was seeing my doctor twice a week. I was beginning to get my energy back, but I was still under hospital care and on a lot of medication. As I was getting better, my mother went back to her shopping. Both of my closets were full of clothes. I couldn't even open of my closets because she had so much stuff inside. It didn't stop her because it was her enjoyment. I didn't want her to feel as if she was putting her life on hold just for me.

However, it got to the point that we begin to get into a lot of arguments for small little things. She realized that I was getting my strength back, and she was ready to go home. She had so much stuff that there were no way she was going to leave them behind. Most of her newly purchased items were for her house. I watched my mother drag her box of items down two flights of stair, and I realized where I got so much of my determination from. I thought how *determined* I was when I dragged my television down three flights of stairs. That morning, I dropped her off at the airport and I promised her that I would make sure that I shipped the remaining boxes to her house by UPS.

CONCLUSION

I loved my mother, but I realized that we were better when we were apart. We were too much alike. I was getting much better; I was now only seeing my doctor once a week. I was getting some of my strength back too. I'd decided to take a trip to Florida to see if I needed to bring Lauren back home with me or just let her stay in Florida; she needed stability in her life. I set up my airline ticket to arrive in Florida July 2 returned back on July 10 because I wanted to be there around Lauren's birthday so that we could celebrate together.

I was in denial about my skin and wore a long blue sleeveless summer dress to Florida. My hair was coming back. It was very short, but I wore it natural. I got off the plane and walked through the terminal. I had to take a shuttle to the opposite side of the airport so that I could pick up my luggage.

Once I got my luggage, I took the escalator down toward the entry level, where I saw Mrs. Scott standing by escalator. "Hey, DD," she said.

"Hi, Mrs. Scott," I said. She gave me a hug. I looked around to see if I saw Lauren.

"Where's Lauren?" I asked. She pointed outside where I saw her SUV parked.

"She's in the car with her cousins," she said.

"Oh, okay." I said. As I followed her outside, I saw Lauren sitting in the back seat. I opened the door.

"Hi Lauren," I said.

"Hi," she said.

"Give me hug. I haven't seen you in a while." She reached over the back seat to give me a hug, but I noticed how she stared at me. She didn't know what to say.

Mrs. Scott got into the driver side and started her truck. She turned around and looked back at her grandchildren. "You guys sit down and put your seat belts on," she said. "Dee, have you ate yet?"

"No," I said.

"We were going to stop at Macaroni Grill for lunch."

"Oh—okay," I said.

Once we arrived at the restaurant, we all got out and went inside, where the hostess greeted us and took us to our table. Lauren and her cousins sat across from us at another table. I noticed that Lauren was very over weight. It was as if she was enjoying everything that was on her plate.

After we finished eating, we all got back into the truck and headed toward Mrs. Scott's house. Once Mrs. Scott drove into the driveway and we got out the car, I walked toward the front door. "Dee, there's a frog by the light as you walked toward the door," Mrs. Scott said. I stopped and I hesitated to take another step.

"Why?" I asked.

"So it can catch the flies and bugs if they try to come into the house."

"Oh, okay." As I got closer to the front door, I ran past the light feature.

Once I entered her house, it looked the same except that she had added on additional rooms to the back of her house. "Dee, do you want to lie down for a while?" she asked. I know you probably a little tired.

"If you don't mind, my feet are so swollen," I said.

"I'm going to let you sleep in Lauren's room while you're here," she said. Lauren never came in the room to talk with me. I felt that she was trying to avoid me. I noticed she stayed in the next room with her cousin and they watched cartoons the entire night.

Later on that night, I got up and walked back where Mrs. Scott's new den that outlook and screen outside attached to their patio. As I walked into the den area, I noticed there was a large screen television that stood in a corner. A long sofa that stood against the wall and a round dinner table and chairs that stood in the middle of the room.

"Dee, we're about to go to get some Church's chicken do you want to go?" Mrs. Scott asked.

"Yea sure," I said. I sat there for couple of days as I watched Mrs. Scott feed her grandchildren. They ate Pop-Tart and sodas in the morning. She ordered pizza mostly every night. I began to realize that they basically ate anything they wanted.

While I was there, it mostly rained everyday, and I would sit and watch television or play solitaire on the computer. I eventually showed Mrs. Scott how to play the game, but once she got the hang of it she spent a lot of her time playing it too.*

One of Lauren's cousin and I would sit and talked while Lauren stayed in the bedroom with her cousins. I noticed that Lauren didn't care that much for her cousin, I guess I had that itching feeling that something strange was going on among them but I couldn't put my finger on it quite yet. Lauren would go back and tell Mrs. Scott everything she did but I also realized that my daughter was really running things and she was very spoiled and very sneaky too.

While I was there, Lauren wore a very long shirt with shorts and I noticed Mrs. Scott wore the same including their hair. I thought I was watching an *Austin Powers* movie were Lauren was mini-me but I was really disappointed to see how large my child has gotten because for the longest I couldn't understand how she would spend the summer with her grandparent and come back overweight but now I beginning to understand.

One day, I combed Lauren's hair into a pretty little ponytail rather than having her hair all over the places. After I did her hair, I could tell by the expression on her faces that she wasn't pleased. Afterward, she walked back to her room, but she didn't realize that I was behind her, taking the comb and brush back into the bedroom. As she got closer to her room, she looked at her cousin with disgust on her faces as she grabbed her ponytail and removed the hair band and she threw it to the floor.

Her cousin saw my face, but Lauren at the time was unaware that I was standing behind her until she turned around. She was shocked, and she could tell that I was pissed. "I don't know who you think you are but you better get yourself together quick," I said. She began to back up as I got closer.

"I'm still your mother, and you will respect me," I said. Don't you play with me or underestimate me because I will spank your behind. She stood there knowing that I wasn't playing. Mrs. Scott was in the other room playing solitaire on the computer.

"What going on Dee?" she asked. I turned around toward the bedroom as I stared back at Lauren.

"I just combed Lauren's hair and I guess she didn't like the way I did it so she took her hair apart and threw the hair band on the floor." I said.

She didn't say anything, but I knew then that even though I had a long way to go to get myself back on my feet I knew my daughter needed to come home. I didn't like what I was seeing. She didn't seem like the same child that I sent to Florida.

It was still raining in Florida. The sun would come out for a while, but later on that day, it would rain. I slept a lot while I was there,

DETERMINATION

but when I was awake, I kept noticing Lauren and her cousin ate junk food throughout the day.

Lauren stayed in the next room with the door closed. I noticed she really didn't care that much for her cousin.

Lauren came in the den and sat on the sofa for a while, pretending she was watching music videos, as I sat talking to her cousin Rachel about what type of music she liked. Lauren got up and left. I was beginning to build a good relationship with Rachel because she was able to open up to me. I thought she was very pretty girl who had a difficult life and all she wanted was someone to love and accept her. I thought she had such a warm and sweet personality, but I could tell something was going on between her and my daughter, but I didn't know what.

As we sat talking, she told me that because Lauren had gained so much weight her grandmother gave her Lauren's old clothes to wear but she didn't think Lauren liked her for that. "Before you got here Miss Robinson, your daughter and I got into a fight," she said.

"You did," I said. She was about to go into details Lauren walked into the door as she listen in the kitchen.

I wasn't sure if she heard us talking but she turned back around and left the room. I decided to follow her, but she didn't know I was right behind her. She walked into the bedroom where I slept as Mrs. Scott played solitaire. Lauren kneeled down to whisper in Mrs. Scott's ear. Lauren turned around with shock on her face once she saw me.

"What's wrong?" I asked. She didn't say anything. Mrs. Scott turned around.

"Oh nothing's wrong," Mrs. Scott said.

Lauren stood looking me straight in my face. I kept eye contact with her letting her know that I knew what she was up to. I went back to the den to talk with Rachel. "Ms. Robinson, you need to move your daughter back home with you," she said. I shuck my head agreeing with her. "Baby, I agree with you," I said. I'm beginning to see what's really going on around here.

The next day we decided to go to the mall. We walked around for a while until we all stopped at a store where there were a lot of creative and fun things that kids could learn and explore about nature in general. I noticed that Lauren was carrying this one item in her hand as she walked around the store though not once was she willing to come up to me and ask would I purchase it for her.

I stood there waiting as she looked over at me from a distant, I ignored her; I was still disappointed how she was acting toward me—and her cousin. I stood there wondering would she ever trust me again

The day of her birthday, I woke up that morning and noticed Lauren wasn't there, but her other cousins were. They were standing in the kitchen. "Where's Lauren?" I asked. Mrs. Scott came out of her room.

"Dee, she went over Bernice's houses," she said.

"But this is her birthday," I said. You would've thought she stayed around for her birthday. I especially came down here to be with her. I started to cry.

"Let us talk in the other room, Dee," she said. I followed her back into her bedroom.

"Mrs. Scott, Lauren needs to come home," I said. She looked at me as if she doesn't notice her own mother. Mrs. Scott walked over to give me a hug. At this time, her younger son walked into the room.

"What's wrong?" he asked Mrs. Scott.

"Oh nothing," she said. "Go back in the kitchen. Let me talk with Dee alone."

"Mrs. Scott, I don't like what I'm seeing here," I said. "My own child doesn't even want to come around me."

"Dee, Lauren is fine you just need to give her some time," she said.

"Mrs. Scott, I don't like what I see. Lauren needs to come home within two weeks."

Out of nowhere, her son walked back into the room. "All we've done for you!" he screamed. "And now you got the nerves to ask for her back!" I looked up at him shocked that he was screaming at me with anger in his voice, which I became afraid.

"Walter don't you say anything else!" Mrs. Scott said. "Let me speak with Dee alone." He kept looking at me.

"You black Mongolian!" he screamed. I got even scared because he was a big guy and he was stood at least six feet tall as he stood there screaming and sweating as he was swallowing three bags of BC Powder down his throat.

"Leave out right now!" she screamed.

"Momma, all we did for Lauren and she wanted to take her back to Texas," he said.

"Leave!" she screamed. Right now!

As I turned back to face her I thought to myself *if she did this unconditionally and she said that they was there to help me then why was he so dramatic? Why wouldn't I want my child back with me?* I told her that I might have let her stay, but after I saw how spoiled and disrespectful she was, I knew then that she needed to come home.

"Dee, she'll come around it has been awhile since she saw you and she has to get adjusted," she said. I stood there in her bedroom and for the first time I saw Mrs. Scott for who she really was. I realize that I really didn't mean that much to her but I had something she wanted and it was my child.

She had manipulated and conned me with her lies just to get what she wanted. There was a lot of good about her but she was selfish when it came to her own family bond. I noticed that she comes off as if she's innocent and she has my best interest at heart. I thought she liked to keep peace among Joseph and myself but she played a major role behind the scenes by keeping up the confusion.

I went back into the den. I sat on the sofa as I watched television. Rachel came and sat next to me. I was very quiet. "Ms. Robinson?' she said.

"Yes," I said.

"You need to get your child," she said.

"What do you mean?" I asked.

"You need to take her back with you."

"Why?" You said that before. But before she could answer, Mrs. Scott came into the room and we both became quiet.

"Dee, you want breakfast?" she asked. I'm fixing something for everyone.

"Sure," I said.

It was still raining. The sun would come out for a while but an hour later, it started raining again but later that day Lauren came home and we celebrate her birthday in the den. Mrs. Scott bought her everything she basically wanted. Clothes, music box with various cases of CDs, a beautiful necklace with a diamond dolphin, a set of Victoria Secret products including a cake that not including yearly passes to Disneyland, MGM, etc.

As we watched, Lauren open her presents, and we thought the presents were very nice. As she looked at her Victoria Secret cases, I said, "That's nice Lauren."

She looked at her grandmother. "But I wanted purple," she said.

"It's the thought that count Lauren," her cousin said.

I gave Lauren this look like you knew better. I just stared at her. I knew she needed to come home because I saw enough. Lauren was very ungrateful and especially disrespectful toward me also.

After she opened her present she left behind a mess after unwrapping her gifts. "Lauren don't you want to pick some of this stuff up and unplug your music box if you're going back to your room?" I asked.

She unplugged the radio and she left out of the room as Rachel and I picked up the wrapping paper. Afterward, we sat and watched television after picking up the mess she left behind. I noticed that Rachel would never go back to that room to play with them; she always sat with me, which I thought it was very polite and sweet of her because she basically kept me company.

"Dee, why don't you and Rachel come and go with me to K-mart." Mrs. Scott said.

"Okay," I said.

We got up and we drove with her to the store. Once we got into the parking lot Mrs. Scott tried to find a parking space. "What were you trying to get Lauren to do earlier?" Mrs. Scott asked. I sat there trying to think about what she was talking about.

"Oh!" I said. Um, I told her that she needed to help us pick up the wrapping paper and if she wasn't listening to her CD player she need to unplug it if she was going back to her room. Why you ask?

"It's really nothing but when she's at my house she can leave whatever she likes on the floor," she said. You don't have to worry about her using up my electricity in my house she's fine. Rachel looked at me as I looked back at her but I didn't say a word because I knew my child needed to come home.

Before I got on the airplane head back to Dallas, I made it clear that Lauren was coming home. I knew Mrs. Scott was disappointed and so was Lauren but I didn't care not after what I saw that week. I knew if I didn't get her back with me now, there was no way I could put some moral values and respect for others. She needed to learn how to appreciate and love God and herself first if she expects others to do the same. It was obvious she was running things in Florida but she definitely won't run things in Texas.

Once I got back to Texas, I made plans for her arrival. I enrolled her into middle school for the coming fall semester. I went to the grocery store and I purchase over $200.00 worth of groceries because I wanted to make sure that there was enough food for both of us.

When I picked her up from the airport, she was happy to see me. She was a different person when she got off that plane because she was very humble and much nicer but she was still a little distant which still bothered me.

When we got home and I opened her luggage as usual, she didn't have any decent clothes to wear which I saw the clothes that she brought her on her birthday that wasn't in her suitcase.

"Lauren where's the clothes that Mrs. Scott brought you on your birthday when I was down there?" I asked.

"I don't know," she said. When it was time for me to come back to Texas, she had hidden my things from me—even my own CDs.

"Really—huh," I said. That's interesting. "Well, I need to take you shopping this weekend because you need clothes for school."

I was still weak from the bone marrow transplant. I told Lauren if she wanted to sleep with me she could but if she wanted to sleep on the sofa she could. "I'll sleep on the couch," she said. "I want to watch TV."

"Oh okay," I said. "I'll see you in the morning then."

When I woke up and I went into the kitchen to start breakfast as I open the refrigerator door. I couldn't believe my eyes. Half of the food was gone. My mouth was open as I slowly closed the refrigerator door as I glanced over at Lauren while she sat watching television.

"Lauren, baby?" I said.

"Yes," she said. Did you eat all this food up like this?

"Yes," she said.

I didn't say anything. I just went back into my bedroom and I sat down thinking that I need to stop her from this cycle because it's

DETERMINATION

going to eventually hurt her in the end because I didn't want her to grow up and have a very low self-esteem about herself.

Later on that day, one of my friends asked if I wanted to have lunch with her, but I had to take Lauren shopping. I asked her if she likes to go with us; we could have lunch afterward, which she was fine with it.

That afternoon she drove us to the Galleria Mall. I took Lauren to Gap to purchase a few items for school. I asked the salesperson for assistance because I didn't know her exact size even though Mrs. Scott told me that Lauren wore a size nine.

Once the guy came from the fitting room, he told me that my daughter wore a size fourteen to sixteen.

"A what," I said.

"She's a size fourteen to sixteen, ma'am," he said. I looked at my friend and she shucks her head.

"But she just turned twelve years old," I said. "I wear a size fourteen to sixteen."

Lauren came back from the fitting room. "Baby, momma has to start watching what you're eating, okay," I said.

"Okay," she said.

After we finish school shopping, we decided to go downstairs to the restaurant to eat lunch. We placed our orders with the waiter while we sat out on the patio area talking until they brought out our food.

Janet and I ordered a salad while Lauren ordered a cheese steak sandwich with fries. The sandwich was so large that it filled the hold plate. Once the waiter brought our food out, I saw Lauren pick up half of her sandwich. Seconds later, as I turned around from talking with my friend, Lauren had the other half of her sandwich in her hands.

Janet stopped eating with her mouth open before I knew it I grabbed her hand before she could put it in her mouth. "No, stop," I said. We can take it home and you can eat it later. Eat your fries.

What have I done? I thought. If I didn't put a stop to this she'll have bad habit of eating when she isn't hungry because she was going to have a difficult time because I was putting on weight myself which I knew I needed help with because I was in menopause but I figure we could try to lose it together which I was gaining non-stop.

Once I got Lauren settled in I begin to get threats from Joseph because the California attorney's office was trying to get him to pay child support which I noticed Mrs. Scott was constantly calling me every since the courts has been pressuring her son.

After speaking with Lauren, she always wanted to talk with me afterward, which I tried to dodge her by being too busy to come to the phone because I felt that she was fishing for information.

But I was getting frustrated with her because I realized that she wasn't as innocent as she portrayed herself to be because if she wanted to keep peace she wouldn't be right in the middle of this ordeal that I was having with her son.

Mrs. Scott supported her son when she knew he wasn't doing right by his daughter. Her family had a very strong bond. I felt she knew her son wasn't doing right by Lauren, but she kept it among them. My mother was different. If we were wrong, she told us no matter who was at fault. She taught us dignity and respect for others and ourselves.

I decided to call my mother because it was beginning to be too much for me to handle. I just didn't want to go through these threats and the harassment as I did in the past.

"Hello," she said.

"Momma, I can't do this anymore." I cried.

"What's wrong?" she asked.

"Momma, Mrs. Scott is calling me a lot because they trying to get Joseph to pay child support."

"Dee, you have to calm down." The next time she calls, you pull out your Bible and read Psalm 37 to her.

"Okay."

So I took my mother's advices. I put my Bible next to the phone because I wanted to be prepared whenever she called which eventually she did call. I wanted this to stop so I took my mother's advices. One day she called wanting to speak to Lauren but I knew she wanted to talk to me. "Hi, Mrs. Scott," I said.

"How you're doing?" she asked

"I'm fine," I said.

"You want to talk to Lauren?"

"Yea let me speak with her."

"Lauren, your grandmother is on the phone, she wants to talk with you," I said. Lauren talked with her for a couple of minutes.

"Momma!" Lauren said.

"Yea," I said.

"My grandmother wants to talk with you." I took the phone.

"Hey," I said.

"I need to see when Lauren can come down to visit?" she asked.

"Not right now," I said. "Mrs. Scott, Lauren isn't a size nine but a size sixteen. I need to get Lauren back to a healthy weight and this fluctuating back and forth is not healthy for her heart."

"I think she looks fine the way she is," she said. The phone went quiet. I took a deep breath.

"Did my son call you today?" she asked.

"Yes," I said. Mrs. Scott, Joseph needs to deal with the courts in California to resolve this matter because he forged my name on those documents. He needs to deal with them.

"But Dee—," she said.

I was getting angry and this conversation wasn't going anywhere. I put the phone on speaker as Mrs. Scott kept talking. I begin to read Psalm 37.

"'Do not fret because of evil men or be envious of those who do wrong; for like the grass they will soon wither, like green plants they will soon die way' (Psalm 31: 1–2)," I said. As she began to scream, I kept reading.

"'Trust the Lord and do good; dwell in the land and enjoy safe pasture. Delight yourself in the Lord and he will give you desires of your heart' (Psalm 31: 3–4)," I said.

After I read majority of the Scripture to her she hung up, but after that day, I decided to move on with my life without Joseph's support. I knew then that someone had to be smart enough to put closure to all this drama because I was tired of all the fighting, which it wasn't getting us nowhere but confusion for Lauren.

I realized that it was time to put more of my faith in God and let him fight my battles and to know that he would always be there for me and my child. He's the head of my household all this time he was there for me and never left my side. I was beginning to put my fears and problems in his hands.

I decided that once Lauren turned eighteen years old she could see her father and his family whenever she wish but I got to get my life together so therefore I can get my child's life on the right track especially when it concerns her health. It took me seven days as it rain in Florida to realize what was really going on but I hope that I'm not too late.

That fall I went back to work part-time and eventually went full-time, but I knew something was wrong because I haven't heard from my mother lately. She usually calls to let me know if everything was okay but something just didn't feel right. I called home and the phone would just ring. I would call and call but nothing I only got her answer machine. I would leave messages but she'll never call back. I called my little sister at work.

"Nicole, where's Momma?" I asked. She's not returning my phone calls.

"Momma is sick, Dee, and she doesn't need to be bothered with you right now," she said.

"What?" I asked. I want to see if she's okay. What's wrong with her, Nicole?

"Dee, the cancer is back," she said.

"What—? Is she going to be okay?" I asked.

"We don't know," she said. My sister was so very dry and to the point that she was unwilling to give me more information on her condition. "Carolyn is with her," she said.

"But she won't pick up the phone," I said.

"Dee, Momma doesn't need to be stressed out," she said. "I got to get back to work, Dee."

I started crying. I couldn't believe that they wouldn't let me talk to Momma. I always felt like an outsider. I felt that I was the last to find out what happens in our family and I couldn't understand that for so long until one of my friends told me, *DD, they can expect of you but you can't expect of them*, which put a lot of my doubts I had in perspective.

I cried many nights hoping that I was able to speak with her. I called again but the phone ringed twice, someone picked up the phone. "Hello—hello," I said. I was shocked when someone answered, but I noticed that it was my oldest sister.

"Carolyn, where's Momma?" I asked.

"Dee, Momma doesn't want to be bothered and she doesn't need to be stressed out," she said.

"Carolyn—" the phone hung up.

"What!" I said. *What did I do to be treated this way?* I asked myself.

I couldn't understand why. I called back. She picked the phone up, and we started a screaming match where we couldn't understand what each other were saying. She hung up again. I cried with so much frustration.

I'm all the way in Texas and they were in Alabama, I couldn't afford to fly home because I didn't have the money. I waited an hour. I called back the answer machine came on, but when it beeped for me to leave a message, I responded, "Momma, I wanted to know if you're okay. Momma, Carolyn won't let me talk with you—"

The phone picked up. "Dee?"

"Momma!" I started to cry again. "Momma, are you okay?" I asked.

"It doesn't look good, Dee," she said. "The doctor was too late; the cancer is in my bones."

"Momma—," I cried.

"You got to get alone with your sisters, Dee," she said. "You're going to need each other in the end. You've been through too much, Dee. You don't need to be stressed out because you're just getting back on your feet yourself." She started to cry. "I love you, Dee," she said.

"I love you too, Momma," I said.

"Try to get alone with your sisters, okay?" she asked.

"Okay," I said. I'll check on you later, Momma, okay."

I didn't realize how serious it was. I thought if I fought (which I knew I got my strength from her), she would be okay too. My nephew called me. "Auntie Dee, my momma and auntie Nicole is fighting; you've got to stop them," he said.

"Baby, it not too much I can do because I don't know the full story, and I don't want to get into the middle of that," I said.

"GG is sick, and they're fighting," he said.

"I know baby, but it's nothing I can do, I'm sorry," I said. "I'm in Texas, and they wouldn't listen to me."

He was the first grandchild and my first nephew in our family. He's my favorite, and I loved him so much. My daughter came into my bedroom she told me that she had a dream about momma.

"What did you dream, Lauren?" I asked her.

"I was at the swimming pool and she walked up to me and we sat and talked and she asked me how I liked school," she said.

"Oh really—," I said.

I knew she wanted to see Lauren before she died but I didn't realized how sick my mother was because if I known I would've figure out a way to get home but they kept me away from her when they didn't realized that even though we couldn't get alone in the same room we loved each other so much and we shared something that was so deadly and that was cancer and we could relate to one another the effects of being sick and being so close to death.

The next day I got a call telling me to come home because Momma had passed away. I didn't know what to think nor what to do I just hope they would prolong her funeral because I didn't want to say good-bye. She was my mother, and the only mother I had but I knew eventually I had go back home and face my fears.

I thought about how other people would come up to me and tell me how proud she was of me, but she never told me herself but once. I wanted so much to make her and my father so proud of me. I guess I wanted their acceptance so badly, but I knew deep inside that they were proud of me already.

"I was the one child she didn't have to worry about," she once said. I was the one who would get up in the morning on the weekend clean the hold house up, wash and hang the clothes outside on the line to dry while she went to yards sales. She use to yell when she couldn't find something but I was the one who use to jump up trying to help her because I wanted so much to show her that I loved her. I guess I just wanted to please them both, but as I got older, I realized they were gone and that was it.

When I finally went home for the funeral, I went to the funeral home to view her body I was sick to my stomach as we walked in. At first, we passed her body as we walked in, but I kept telling my friend that's my mother. She was a little dark in the face from all the chemotherapy but I knew that it was her.

We walked back and we sat down as family came in but I was at peace with my mom before she died. I didn't leave or regret not telling her how much I loved her. I knew that I was her daughter, her protector and as I wrote this book things became so clearer to me because we were so much alike because we love from our hearts and we are so easy to forgive and I wouldn't change anything because she have given me so much determination to fight as my father was so motivating and I will love them for the rest of my life.

I was still in denial about my skin when I went back to work. I wore skirts but I gradually start wearing pants. My shirts were normally long sleeves or mid-sleeves. I couldn't wear anything strapless because of the surgical scar on my chest. Even if I wore a v-neck shirt, I sewed up the v-neck a little so that the scar wouldn't be so noticeable or I'll use *Derma blend* products to cover the scar.

It was an adjustment for me when it came to my skin because I was use to wearing short sleeves shirts, dresses, skirts, or shorts but not anymore. I was too ashamed for others to see my skin or my body because I was so afraid they would ask me questions, which I felt that I had to go into details about my prognoses.

I decided that I needed to start working out. I decided to join the gym down stair at my job, which I didn't feel comfortable undressing in front of others. I would go into one of the stalls in the bathroom to undress because I tried once but I was still embarrassed that people would notice.

I took baths at night because whenever I took a shower or bath in the morning my skin would get so dry I would ach or itch with so much pain that tingled through my legs and sometime my arms. I had to sit on the edge of my bed or I lie across the bed crying sometimes until the pain went away.

I didn't feel comfortable unless I was at home behind closed doors. I was so insecure about my body that I never forgot that I was given a second chance in life but I begin to think about others who probably had the same problem that I was going through so I decided to find out if there were other options to change the way my skin looked.

I set up an appointment with various dermatologists. At first when I went in to see doctors, I explained to them my prognoses and how it discolored my skin. I was so emotional because I was ashamed that I had to take my clothes off but eventually they stated that it wasn't too much they could do for me.

One doctor gave me medicated cream and foam to use but nothing. I even went on various Web sites looking for something natural to use for the discoloration which I found this foam but it didn't help. I thought that maybe I had vitiligo because some of the patches on my body were a very pale color.

I decided to do more research on various dermatologists in Dallas area that handle vitiligo patients, but at the time, I had to take Lauren in to see a dermatologist for her acne. I also set up an appointment for myself too because I wanted to see if he could recommend a doctor that could probably help me locate someone that deals with vitiligo.

There were two doctors we saw that day one doctor visited with my daughter and the other one visit with me. When I pulled my pants leg up so that he could see my scars, he explained to me that it wasn't anything his office could do but he knew a doctor that specialized with vitiligo patients.

"Are you sure your skin wasn't like this all your life?" he said. "Even before you had a bone marrow transplant?"

"No," I said.

"Are you sure?"

"Yes sir, my skin was fine until I had the bone marrow transplant."

"Well okay then, if you say so," he said. Shock was all over my faces because I felt that he didn't believe me. He gave me a piece of paper with this doctor's name and phone number on it.

"Call him," he said. And see if he can help you. He stays booked up but I think he will be able to tell you more than I can, okay.

"Okay."

"Why don't you follow me," he said. "Let's see how your daughter is doing." I got up from the patient table and I followed him to the other room. He opened the door.

"Excuse me, young lady, let me ask you a quick question?" he asked my daughter. "Have your mother skin always been this way?" My daughter had hesitation on her face because she didn't know what to say.

"I don't know," she said. My mouth was open I was shock because if anyone should have known it would've been her.

"Ms. Robinson, it was nice meeting you, and I'm sorry there wasn't much I could do," he said.

"Oh—that's fine," I said. He left out the room and closed the door where I stood watching the other doctor assistant my daughter.

The doctor looked back at me to tell me what type of medicated cream he would recommend for my daughter's skin, but he noticed that I had tears in my eyes. He didn't say anything; he kept assisting Lauren.

After we left the doctor's office, we walked in the parking lot toward my car. Lauren knew I was angry because I didn't say much as we got into the car.

"Lauren, why you didn't defend me?" I asked. She just sat there with her mouth open.

"Lauren?' I said.

"I don't know—," she said.

"Lauren, if anyone should know me, it should've been you."

She still didn't say anything. I sat there trying to calm my nerves because I was really frustrated because I was getting the same results each time from every dermatologist. As I looked into my hands, I noticed the paper with the doctor's name and number who handled vitiligo patients. As we sat in the car, I decided to call the doctor's office to set up me an appointment. I scheduled to see him next month because he was booked up until then. *He must be a good doctor,* I thought.

A month later I went to Southwestern Medical Center to visit with the doctor but once they called me to the back the doctor's nurse asked me what was my purpose of coming in which I explained my condition to her which she seems to be aware of the symptom. She asked me to get fully undress as she provided me a gown that wrap from the back.

"Dr. Whitley should be in to see you soon," she said. Ten minutes later the doctor walked in with his nurse.

"Hello my name is Dr. Whitley," he said. What can I do for you today?

"I had a bone marrow transplant back in February of 98," I said. But it left my skin with a lot of discolorations all over my body.

"Let me see?" he asked. As he touched and rubbed my skin, he begins to touch my upper arm.

"Your skin is so soft," he said. Most bone marrow patient skin is normally hard after the procedure. I think we should use the PUVA procedure."

"What's that?" I asked.

"We basically exposed your body with ultraviolet light for severe skin diseases but first we will give you this medication that's light sensitive with a combination of ultraviolet light which would help bring color back in your skin," he said.

"I think it would probably take at least six months, but we first need to take before and after pictures so that we can put them in your files for references," he said. I will have one of our assistance shows you the unit and while we'll check to see if you're insurance would cover this procedure.

"Thank you," I said.

I was so happy and very excited that I finally found someone who could help me when it came to my skin. Before I left their assistant took me into this small room where there was a large round object standing at least six feet tall in the middle of the room. She begins to explain to me what the object was. "This is a UVB light unit," she said. As she opened the door, I looked inside where I notice a lot of bulbs. "We call these ultraviolet lights," she said. They are large and long light bulbs which deliver UV light to your skin.

As I looked into the cabinet, there were light bulbs that surrounded the hold unit. "Your treatment could last anywhere from a minute to thirty minutes," she said. We have to see how much your insurance would cover first but you need to see ophthalmology before the procedure because the Oxsoralen medication can develop cataract in your eyes.

She handed me these forms that the ophthalmology had to fill out during my examination. I noticed there were tips for dry skin, which it explained that I needed to bath or shower for ten to fifteen minutes. Use lukewarm, not hot water, minimize the use of soap especially to dry areas which it went on to say that I need to pat dry not rub my skin and leave some moisture on my skin.

Once I found a ophthalmologist in my area, I explained to him why I needed my eyes examine which he told me that he has to give me a full examination which I was fine with but I stayed there for over four hours until he dilate my eyes. He was still unwilling to sign off on the forms until I came back for more tests.

When I went back for more test he only provide my contacts which I was hopeful that he would sign the examination form but stated he only had time for fitting of my contacts which took five minutes which he charged me one hundred dollars for even though my insurance company also paid him.

I was pissed but I knew I couldn't go back there I decided to go onto the Internet where I was able to find a dermatologist that dealt with patients who has or have Graft vs. Host Disease (GVHD). I found a doctor that was located in North Dallas at the Texas Dermatology Association. I called to set up an appointment to meet with her, which she was very familiar with my disease once we meet.

She made a suggestion that rather than me doing PUVA procedure she thought that it would be best to try the Narrowband procedure but she wanted to first check with her head nurse who handled all the procedure to see which one was the best PUVA or the Narrowband which she suggested the Narrowband.

The doctor wanted me to come into the office three times a week. I met with the nurse afterward where she showed me the full body cabinet where there were light fixtures inside the panels. I noticed the name on the cabinet, which stated National Biological Corporation HOUVA II. Every Monday, Wednesdays and Fridays of each week I was scheduled to come in the morning.

My first day I didn't know what to expect but I was insecure about my body as I waited for them to call me to the back room. The nurse showed me what I needed to do. "Okay, you need to take off all your clothes except for your panties. You can pull them off when you get inside. There are sunglasses by the wall that you need to put on your eyes before we start the procedure," she said.

"Okay," I said.

"Once you're finish with sunglasses you need to put them in the other tray so that they can be cleaned."

"Okay."

"Did you bring your pillowcase?" she asked.

"Yes, I brought two," I said.

"Okay once you're finish put your pillowcase with your name on your bag and put them in one of the open shelves, okay, she said. Once you've ready knock on the door and one of us would come in.

"Okay." I said. Thank you. I got undressed; I put the dark sunglasses on with the pillowcases in my hand as I knocked on the door. I rushed into the cabinet before one of them entered the room.

The nurse came into the room. "Are you ready?" she asked.

"Yes," I said. I covered my body with the pillowcases, as she got closer to me because I was too embarrassed but it seems as if she was familiar with patients who had these similar problems with their skin.

She closed the cabinet door as she looked through the open window. "Ms. Robinson, you need to take off your panties," she said.

"Okay," I said. I pulled them off. She begins to key in numbers as the light came on and the warm breeze air came from underneath my feet.

That first time I was in there for at least a minute, I put my clothes on and I left but eventually the more I came the more minutes I stayed in the cabinet. I came faithfully three times a week during my lunch hours. Eventually I was down to Monday and Friday. I begin to see a different in my skin I was so shock.

Now, I was down to once a week. The doctors told me that seventy percent of my skin was back but it has been almost two years now I was still going through the procedure. I wanted to see more improvement in my skin which I begin to feel more positive and confidences in myself again.

I knew I probably wouldn't get my skin back to it natural color but as long as it help me build my self-esteem up I was willing to take a chances so that maybe someone who might be going through the same can have a chances to feel human again and not be ashamed to wear various type of clothes without drawing unwanted attention. Eventually my doctor diagnosed me with Trichrom Vitiligo.

It has been ten years since I was diagnose with Leukemia but as I wrote this book, I've learned so much about myself where I'm able to move on with my life. I've learned how to forgive and to see things in different way so that I'm able to grow and think outside the box.

When it's all said and done I've learned how to embraces our differences meaning my family, Joseph's family and others but in a respectful way because we're all God's children and we're different for a reason so that we can learn and respect one another.

DETERMINATION

After my mother's death, I wrote my donor to tell her how thankful I was because I was amazed that she was on the National Registry because of the percentage is very low to locate for African American donors and how I felt blessed that she was on there which she saved my life.

My doctors told me that I couldn't see my donor until a year after the procedure. They didn't want the donor to feel sad or guilty if I became ill or died between the times she donated her marrow to me. I sent pictures, my address and phone number just in cases she wanted to meet me. She eventually wrote me back:

Dear Recipient,

It was wonderful to hear from you. It was in honors that I went on the National Bone Marrow list. It was a great pleasure and tribute to the two women I love the most to try to help another human being. We speak of you often and I hope you continue to do well.

The wonderful people at the American Red Cross are great about keeping me informed on your progress. Hopefully we will have the opportunity to meet one another. It would be fun and joyful. My family has remained firmly behind my decision to move forward with the donation. They are firm in their belief that we do what we can, within our limitations to help someone else survive cancer. They continue to be in your corner.

I do not know how much you have been told about me but I'm not a minority, which makes the miracle of our connection only more special. God must have wonderful plans for you if he crossed racial lines to give you a new opportunity for life. It has been my privilege and pleasure to be part of something so special.

Please continue to stay in touch, you continue to remain in my daily thoughts and prayers

Your special friends

Deagara Robinson

I was so happy that I heard from her. But I was also shocked that she wasn't of my race after I read her letter. I felt blessed that she was willing to save my life because she loved unconditionally. She went the extra mile to save my life even though she didn't know who I was. I love her and I know one day I'll see my additional family but I knew I had to do this book first because I was the lucky one. There are so many people who are still waiting and searching for a donor and there are some who have died waiting.

I was at the North Park mall one Saturday and there was a table set up asking people to register to become bone marrow donor. I stopped by and I told them that my bone marrow recipient and my donor was an unrelated donor but I haven't heard back from her after I sent her letters. He told me that maybe she doesn't want to be found and that it was best to leave it alone. I became very teary eyed as I walked away feeling empty inside but I thought maybe he's right but I wanted her to know how thankful I am for giving me a second chances in life.

You have people like my donor who was willing to open their hearts, souls, and minds to save lives without knowing who they are. My struggles living with Leukemia has changed me into a better person. I want to help others understand what it's like to have this disease. This is not about me anymore. This is about changing peoples thought and beliefs about Leukemia through my eyes. Just maybe there are others who are willing to do the same but unsure what would be the outcome or if they're unaware how dangerous this disease really is but a bone marrow transplant saves lives. I was unaware until it came knocking at my door.

My life was very hard and I know that. But I wanted to share my story and to also bring some type of knowledge about Leukemia because I've experience it personally. But I've learned that with consistency, determination and unconditionally love you can save lives and it really feels good when you can give back. I want to give back because she gave me back my life why should I not try to save others.

I've grown to feel the suffering and the loss of others and maybe it had to take me to go through this challenge in my life to see things in a different perspective and just learn how to love others for who they are because we're all God's children and some of us have to go through our trial and tribulation to grow so that it can make us even stronger and to become a better person within ourselves.

I've learned through determination that I could take something that was so negative in my life and change it into something positive so that I could grow and maybe help others to believe and to hope again. There are so many people in this world that is or has been in worse predicaments than I have but I've learned that we're not perfect and that God sometimes bring things to us to make us stronger so that we can learn how to handle situations in a better way.

I know that I've said and done some things that I wish I could take back but I've learn to apologize and to accept my mistakes and move on. It takes a bigger person to say that they're sorry and really mean it. We all make mistakes but we sometime let our pride get in our way. If we can sometime say what we really feel from our hearts, we can have a better understanding of ourselves and acknowledge that whatever particular issues we made in the past we need to learn how to faces our own fears and mistakes head on which I have.

I'm at peace with myself. I held onto so much anger that now I realized that I've changed. When Mrs. Scott called me at work back in May 2004, Lauren was about to graduate from high school. When she called me at work, I was shocked because I haven't spoken to her for six years so basically I was caught off guard after I read Psalm 37.

"DD, Mrs. Scott, is on the line." The receptionist said.

"Okay," I said. I picked up the phone

"Hello, Mrs. Scott," I said. How you're doing?

"I'm fine," she said. I'm calling to check on Lauren to see if she's doing fine.

"Oh, she's doing fine," I said. She's graduating in a couple of weeks. But she looks great. She lost all of her weight and she's pretty as ever.

"Uh huh," she said sarcastically. The phone went silent.

"Well she looked fine the way she was," she said. I took a deep breath because I knew nothing had changed.

"Mrs. Scott, I told Lauren when she turns eighteen years old that she can visit you guys whenever she likes because I couldn't stop her from seeing you because she'll be up in age where she could make her own decisions," I said.

I could tell that she was getting angry with me so I told her that I had to go which we hung up. But within thirty minutes, there was a voice message left on my phone at work, it was Joseph but he left me a direct and dry message telling me to have Lauren call him. I decided to call him back to explain to him what I told his mother.

"Hi, Joseph, I've received your voice message," I said.

"I need you to have Lauren to call me," he said. I know her graduation is coming up.

"To be honest, Joseph I know you probably want to attend her graduation but I don't think it's best right now for you to come," I said. She's doing great and I don't want her to see us get into any argument.

"Plus you haven't supported her in the past. I told your mother that when Lauren turns eighteen years old she's welcome to have a relationship with you guys. I just don't want to fight with you guys anymore," I said.

"When she gets away from you I'm going to tell her how evil you are and she's going to see the real you," he said.

"Well, if you feel that way—go ahead, I'm not fighting anymore," I said.

"I hate you!" he screamed.

"What?" I asked.

"I hate your guts!" he said.

"I don't hate you," I said.

"You're evil, and once you die with cancer, I'm going tell our daughter about the real you."

"If you feel that you have to then go ahead. That not going to change things."

"That's why you're going to die," he kept saying.

"We're all going to die one day, Joseph."

"I hate you."

"I don't hate you. I really don't, but I'll pray for you." I said.

"That's why your mother is dead," he said.

"Yea, unfortunately she died, but I still love her, and I don't hate you or wish that on your mother either, but we got to stop fighting for Lauren sake," I said.

He started crying, and he began to scream. I was unable to understand what he was trying to say, but at the same time, he couldn't get to me because I realized then that I've moved on and I've changed. I was really sorry that I hurt him to the point that he hated me so much. But it's too late for me to dwell on the past because this hand was dealt to me but it was up to me on how I was going to handle this and for me to take a hard look at myself.

I had the utmost respect for Mrs. Scott because she was there for me. But God had to open my eyes where I was able to stand up for what I believe in because I had it bad for wanting to make everybody happy and I didn't want them to be angry with me but in the end I was the one that was unhappy but not anymore.

I couldn't write this book until I was honest with myself and what I believe in my heart where I'm able to share a part of me. I knew I had to "Clean my own house." Meaning I can't make judgments on others when I haven't taken a closer look at me? I made the decision to leave my child down with Mrs. Scott she didn't force me to do that but at the same time I knew she wanted the best for Lauren because she loved her.

My mother tried to warn me but I didn't want to listen to her. She saw this but I was so stubborn because I thought I was doing the right thing. I was young and naive about life in general. I put a lot my trust in others but I realized that some would eventually turn on me because I wasn't willing to observe the important things in life because I wasn't patient enough.

I miss my parents and I'll never be able to call my mom to say hello or to say "I love you and that I'm sorry for being so hard headed." Or to tell my father to forgive me for not recognizing him for the good things he tried to teach us when we were younger.

My parents played a major role in my life. I only have memories now. If they weren't concern about some of the decisions I made my life then I would've felt that they really didn't love me. I felt blessed to have shared the wonderful times we did have together as a family.

I see so much of my father in my brother when it comes to his determination to keep us grounded and together as a family. He's our foundation now and I understand his heart because we are so much like our parents and sometime I want so much to protect him but I know that's not my job so I pray and thank God, he's in our lives.

Someone told me once that God was a selfish God and that I should put him first in my life, which I have. At first I thought was selfish but not anymore. I know now that's it smarter to listen rather being too quick to respond. Now, I want to be able to relate with others and understand what that person might be going through or went through in their lives. I want to be able to relate with a person that can talk to me rather than talking at me because I know then if they're really listening and understand what I might be feeling and vice versa.

But in the end, I thank God that he blessed me with so much

wisdom and he brought some of the most positive people in my life because as I got older and as I wrote this book I have a clear understanding of myself and where my faith should be. I've learn how to let God fight my battles for me and to learn how to love a person by how you wanted to be treated.

I'm a better person for myself because I'm much stronger spiritually within where I can love a person unconditionally. I've asked God to keep me humble because I'm not trying to portray myself as if I'm better than the next person, but we have choices and he has given us so much knowledge about ourselves so that we can grow within. I'm a true believer in dreaming for your goals because God put them there for a reason because life is too short.

When I thought that there was no hope for my discoloration in my skin, I didn't give up. I kept searching. I cried plenty times but my conscious and my determination kept me striving to find someone that would be able to help me but as I look back I have so much respect for my doctors especially the one that I thought didn't have good bedside manner. He had them but he knew that he couldn't tell me what I wanted to hear because he didn't really know if I was going to live or die that wasn't his position to give me false hope. I've learn that in his quiet and gracious way he saved my life.

It takes courage to face our fears and I'm proud of who I am because God has created me and he wouldn't bring something on me that he knew I couldn't handled. I sometime feel that some of us as African American don't try to lift each other up in a positive way because we are sometime afraid of the unknown where we are able to face our own fears because when there's knowledge there's hope.

We praise God but some of us aren't willing to take the time to save ourselves or others until it hits home? Until someone in their family they love dearly has been diagnose with Leukemia. The only way to prolong his or her life is with a bone marrow transplant but you find there's not enough minorities on the registry so it give less hope for surviving.

I did something very selfish as I look back. When I was in the hospital most of my white friends called wanting to know where they could go to get tested as my donor, I told them they couldn't because the proteins in our bodies were different but I thought *why I didn't tell them to go in for others who was waiting to find a donor?* Today it haunts me because my donor wasn't a minority. My donor almost lost someone who is so dear to her heart. If she wasn't on the registry twelve years before my diagnoses, I wouldn't be here today.

Life is a struggle, but I don't wear God on my sleeves, and I don't have to shout to the world of my belief in God because he's in my heart, my soul, and my spirit. I thank him for giving me a second chance in life, and I hope by me writing this book and sharing my struggle hopefully it will give you hope too.

listen|imagine|view|experience

AUDIO BOOK DOWNLOAD INCLUDED WITH THIS BOOK!

In your hands you hold a complete digital entertainment package. Besides purchasing the paper version of this book, this book includes a free download of the audio version of this book. Simply use the code listed below when visiting our website. Once downloaded to your computer, you can listen to the book through your computer's speakers, burn it to an audio CD or save the file to your portable music device (such as Apple's popular iPod) and listen on the go!

How to get your free audio book digital download:

1. Visit www.tatepublishing.com and click on the e|LIVE logo on the home page.
2. Enter the following coupon code:
   a75d-ff2b-4ce2-eb41-4811-a2cd-2e3b-79f8
3. Download the audio book from your e|LIVE digital locker and begin enjoying your new digital entertainment package today!